Silicone Survivors

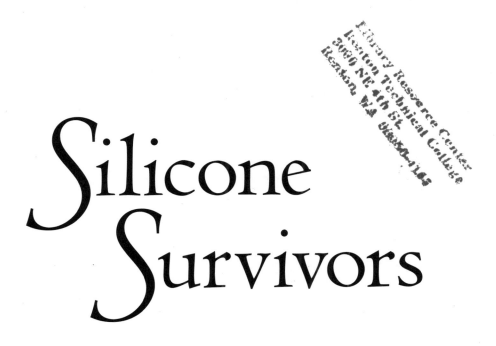

Silicone Survivors

Women's Experiences with Breast Implants

Susan M. Zimmermann

 Temple University Press
PHILADELPHIA

Temple University Press, Philadelphia 19122
Copyright © 1998 by Temple University.
All rights reserved
Published 1998
Printed in the United States of America

⊚ The paper used in this publication meets the requirements of
American National Standard for Information Sciences—Permanence
of Paper for Printed Library Materials, ANSI Z39.48-1984

Library of Congress Cataloging-in-Publication Data

Zimmermann, Susan, 1966–
    Silicone survivors : women's experiences with breast implants /
Susan M. Zimmermann.
        p.   cm.
    Includes bibliographical references and index.
    ISBN 1-56639-611-5 (cl. : alk. paper). — ISBN 1-56639-612-3
(pbk. : alk. paper).
    1. Breast implants—Complications.   2. Silicones—Toxicology.
3. Breast implants—Psychological aspects.   I. Title.
RD539.8.Z56   1998
618.1'90592—dc21   97-45536
                                                           CIP

To those who spoke so openly

Contents

Acknowledgments ix

1 Introduction 1

2 Historical Background: The Emergence of a Controversy 20

3 The Decision to Seek Breast Implants: Women's
Participation in the Medicalization Process 42

4 False Expectations: An Ironic Twist on "Before and After" 70

5 Misinforming Women of Risk: A Medical Conspiracy? 91

6 Minimizing Women's Troubles 115

7 Listening to an Inner Voice 145

8 Transforming Identities: Experiences of Empowerment 169

Notes 191

Bibliography 213

Index 223

Acknowledgments

I could not have completed this book without the support of many people. I particularly wish to thank Phil Brown for suggesting that I look into the breast implant issue, and for his enthusiasm, encouragement, and insightful advice throughout all phases of my research and writing; Lynn Davidman for her friendship, empathy, and constructive criticism of my work; and Susan Bell, for generously giving her time and sharing her resources and knowledge. Susan's own work in the areas of gender, science, and medical innovations influenced my own thinking tremendously. I also thank Susan Allen and Mary Fennell for their helpful suggestions and comments on a later draft of the manuscript, and Calvin Goldscheider, the former Chair of the sociology department at Brown University, for finding funds to subsidize my research travel expenses.

Many other individuals were a constant source for assistance, inspiration, and motivation. Gaelen Benway and Desiree Ciambrone helped me develop a strategy for coding the massive piles of transcripts and fieldnotes I had accumulated, and Judith Kirwan Kelley spent hours helping me locate library resources. A number of friends and colleagues have contributed to this book in other ways, either by supplying me with an endless stream of newspaper clippings and magazine articles, by engaging me in useful discussions related to my work, or by keeping me informed of the most recent scientific studies and publications on breast implants. For these efforts, I especially would like to thank Jeanne

Leffers, Ann Biddlecom, Lori Hunter, Martha Lang, Kristan Schoultz, and Helene Hill.

My family and peers outside of the academic community also have been tremendously helpful and supportive throughout the course of my research. I particularly wish to thank my parents, Albert and Lenore Zimmermann, and my two sisters, Anne Crimmins and Amanda Diffley, for their generosity and ceaseless words of encouragement. I am also grateful to Michael Laidlaw, who, with his background in science, helped me understand and interpret numerous studies on implant-related risk and who, with his love, patience, and sense of humor, has enriched my life in a way that made the completion of this book possible.

I thank Michael Ames at Temple University Press for his sound editorial advice and for engaging in conversations with me about my research before I began piecing together chapters. His enthusiasm for my work at this early stage continued until the manuscript was completed. I am also grateful to Alexa Selph for her excellent copyediting.

I extend my gratitude to the individuals who helped me find women with breast implants to interview. Many of these individuals must remain anonymous since they were participants in this study; however, others need not, including Laurie DeRose, Kat Carter-Stein, and Maura Sheehan. I also thank the organizations that expressed an interest in my work and assisted me with my recruitment efforts, including the American Society of Plastic and Reconstructive Surgeons, the Boston Women's Health Book Collective, the Rhode Island Women's Health Collective, and the numerous support groups for breast implant recipients that placed announcements about my research in their newsletters.

My deepest, heartfelt thanks goes to the forty women I interviewed, who allowed me into their lives, who shared with me their frustrations, suffering, and tears, and who taught me about the irony of their empowerment. For reasons of confidentiality, I have changed the names of all the women who participated in the study, as well as the names of their family members, physicians, attorneys, and friends. I dedicate this book to these women, whose willingness to talk so openly about their experiences with breast implants made this study possible.

Silicone Survivors

1

Introduction

I arrived at Jenna's home at five o'clock on a hot and humid evening in the middle of June 1994.[1] The house was at the end of a street in an affluent suburban neighborhood. Only three other homes occupied the street—one was still under construction. The front yards of the houses appeared newly landscaped; the grass was artificially green, and the shrubs and bushes that lined the front walks were perfectly manicured.

A young girl in a bathing suit with a wet towel draped across her shoulders answered the doorbell. Assuming that the girl was Jenna's daughter, I explained, "Hi, I am Susan. I have a meeting scheduled with your mother." "Hold on a second," the girl replied and disappeared up the hall stairwell. As I stood waiting, two small boys, also in swimsuits, ran around in the downstairs part of the house, laughing and screaming, twirling up their towels and whipping them across each other's legs. Across the room, through a window, I could see a man (probably the children's father) skimming the family's outdoor swimming pool. In less than a minute, the girl who had greeted me returned and in her soft-spoken voice said, "My mother will see you now." I followed her upstairs into her parents' bedroom.

In the large room was a king-size canopy bed and a sitting area consisting of a couple of chairs, a coffee table, and a Victorian-style couch. The curtains in the room had been drawn and the lights dimmed low, providing a quiet and somber atmosphere, a sharp contrast with the lively scene downstairs. With a pillow propped behind her back, Jenna was resting on the couch. "Make yourself comfortable, Susan," she said.

I began setting up my tape recorder while I again explained to Jenna the purpose of our interview. During an earlier phone conversation, I had told her that I was interviewing women who had breast implants; I wanted to understand how they had arrived at the decision to undergo surgery to enhance or reconstruct their bodies, and how having breast implants has affected their lives.

I also explained that I was interested in learning how women with breast implants were coping with medical uncertainty. Since the early 1990s, the media has increasingly disseminated conflicting information about implant-related risk. This publicity began shortly after Mariann Hopkins won a $7.3 million lawsuit against Dow Corning Corporation, the leading manufacturer of breast implants. Hopkins alleged that her own implants had caused her to develop debilitating autoimmune diseases and that Dow had withheld information about these risks from the public prior to her surgery. Although Hopkins won her case, the existence of a relationship between implants and disease has remained the subject of both public and scientific debate. To this day, many physicians and implant manufacturers maintain the view that breast implants are "safe," even though anecdotal evidence suggests that the devices have dangerous side effects. By January 1992, so many implant recipients had reported experiencing implant-related complications and health effects to the Food and Drug Administration (FDA) that the FDA restricted the use of the devices until manufacturers could provide evidence of their safety and efficacy. Although the FDA's decision generated further popular media commentary on the breast implant controversy, I began to notice that there was scant scholarly attention to breast implants outside of epidemiological and medical journals. As a medical sociologist, I told Jenna that I wanted to understand how women themselves were interpreting the conflicting information about implant-related risk, as well as how they felt the medical community was responding to the uncertainty associated with these devices.

Jenna began telling her story. Like many of the women I had previously interviewed, Jenna received breast implants because she was unhappy about the way her breasts appeared after nursing her three children. She explained that her spouse, who was "very fitness- and beauty-conscious," contributed to her poor sense of body image. She was ashamed to undress in front of him and continually made attempts to hide her "stringy and stretched-out" breasts from his view.

In 1989 Jenna decided to visit a plastic surgeon. She told me, "I thought that maybe he could somehow surgically 'lift' the sagging breast tissue." Although Jenna had no intention of receiving breast implants, the surgeon convinced her that he could make her look "as good as new" with these devices. Jenna admitted that the surgery sounded simply "too good to be true," but she trusted her doctor, assuming that physicians were knowledgeable about the risks associated with the procedures they performed and the devices they used. Since her surgeon told her that receiving breast implants was practically "risk-free," breast enhancement seemed like a logical solution for improving her poor self-image. Moreover, Jenna's surgeon provided her with names and phone numbers of his patients who already had received breast implants. When Jenna called these women, they explained that they were "thrilled" with their new bodies, claiming that their husbands thought they "looked beautiful."

What Jenna had thought would be a simple and safe procedure to provide her with a new appearance turned into a nightmare. One month after Jenna received her implants, she had to have them replaced because one had migrated from her chest to her armpit, and both devices caused her breasts to become extremely hard. A year and a half after her replacement surgery, Jenna began to experience a wide range of strange symptoms. First, she developed a rash across her chest and stomach that lasted for over two months, then mysteriously disappeared. Soon after, she began noticing that she was unable to exercise as often as she used to. Prior to receiving implants she ran three miles a day; however, her runs became shorter and less frequent because her knees would swell up and her back and shoulders would ache when she exerted herself. Eventually, Jenna's pains progressed to the rest of her body—she lost mobility in her hips, wrists, and hands. She also began to experience fevers and was bedridden for several days at a time.

Unaware of a potential link between breast implants and autoimmune disease, Jenna could not imagine what was causing her to feel so miserable. She always ate healthy foods and took good care of herself. The doctors she saw all told her that they could find nothing physically wrong with her. With no name for her troubles, Jenna tried to ignore her symptoms and to continue with her daily activities. However, her health began to deteriorate even further. Some days she was so tired and feverish that she could not get out of bed to drive her children to school or prepare their meals. In addition, Jenna noticed that her hair was falling out. As these symptoms progressed, Jenna began to think that something was terribly wrong with her. Not until 1991, however, did she connect her poor health to her implants.

One evening, about two years after Jenna's initial visit to her plastic surgeon, she turned on the television and began watching *Prime Time Live*. To her surprise, the show was airing a segment about the dangers associated with silicone breast implants. On the television screen, a surgeon hovered over a woman's body draped with a blue surgical cloth. With his gloved hands he was scooping out a gooey, slimy gel from the woman's chest and tossing the substance into a metal container adjacent to the operating table. The message the program conveyed was that breast implants can rupture or leak silicone into women's bodies and potentially cause serious autoimmune symptoms and diseases. Jenna was alarmed: Her own plastic surgeon had told her that her breast implants would last forever. Jenna began thinking about her own history of health problems. It all began to make sense to her—prior to receiving breast implants, she had been in good health—after her surgery, her health began to deteriorate.

Despite her worsening symptoms, her physicians dismissed her concerns, telling her that all the scientific studies on implant-related risk indicated that the relationship between breast implants and disease was "not significant." Unable to come up with a diagnosis for Jenna's symptoms, one physician told her that she ought to consider visiting a psychiatrist—that perhaps her real troubles were in her head, not in her body. Jenna eventually found one doctor who was willing to acknowledge the possibility that these devices could be contributing to her poor health. This doctor ordered an X ray of Jenna's breasts, which confirmed that both of her implants had ruptured. Six weeks later, Jenna made the painful decision to have her implants removed.

Even after ex-plantation, Jenna continued to experience a wide range of debilitating symptoms, including chronic fatigue, hair loss, occasional disorientation, and joint pain. More recently she was diagnosed with rheumatoid arthritis.[2] Not only has Jenna's health worsened, but from the multiple surgeries she has undergone, she now has a "massacre" across her chest. Ironically, a procedure that was intended to make Jenna more "beautiful," appear more "feminine," and improve her poor self-image, has left her disfigured and fearful about the future. Even when she is asleep, her dreams remind her of her ordeal: "Every night I have nightmares. . . . Some nights I dream about a woman who has breast cancer and then develops three breasts. Other nights I dream of strippers. And then, some nights I dream that my hair is falling out— that I touch my hair and it will all come out. I just am really bothered, constantly, constantly afraid. I just don't know what the future holds for me."

Experiences and Methodology

This book is an interview-based study of women's experiences with breast implants. It is about how women arrive at the decision to surgically alter or reconstruct a part of their body that is intrinsically linked to ideas about femininity, and about how they come to view this decision after learning that this method of achieving a cultural ideal has either failed, or has the potential to fail. Feminist scholars have noted that, as the most pronounced part of the female body, breasts are a source of female pride and sexual identification, as well as a source of competition, insecurity, shame, and confusion. In the words of the feminist scholar Susan Brownmiller, breasts are "the chief badge of gender."[3] Similarly, the feminist philosopher Iris Young comments, "A woman . . . often feels herself judged and evaluated according to the size and contours of her breasts, and indeed she often is. For her and for others, her breasts are the daily visible and tangible signifier of her womanliness, and her experience is as variable as the size and shape of breasts themselves."[4] Given the meanings attributed to breasts in our culture, what life experiences lead women to turn to plastic surgery for breast implantation? And, if breast size and shape are so intertwined with definitions of femininity and womanhood, how do women with breast implants make sense of their identity as "feminine" if they experience implant-related troubles and complications?

As I answer these questions throughout the pages of this text, I explore the dynamic interplay between cultural assumptions about femininity and societal expectations of medicine and science. In Western culture, medicine and science are presumed to be rational, objective, and value-neutral disciplines that perpetuate a reliance on a simplistic, cause-and-effect model for "treating" and "curing" disease. The logic of this model guides plastic surgeons' practices. For instance, the American Society of Plastic and Reconstructive Surgeons has proclaimed that small breasts are "deformities [that] are really a disease which in most patients result in feelings of inadequacy, lack of self-confidence, distortion of body image and a total lack of well-being due to a lack of self-perceived femininity."[5] The labeling of small breasts as a "disfiguring disease" ("micromastia" is the correct diagnostic label) has led plastic surgeons to believe they can provide any woman who feels inadequate and unfeminine with a quick and simple solution to their troubles—breast implants. In this way, plastic surgeons are capable of creating and perpetuating definitions of ideal female appearances—they decide which female bodies are "diseased" and "in need" of surgical alteration, and with their medical expertise, they are able to mold and reshape women into "perfect" images of femininity.

However, plastic surgeons are not the only ones who participate in the labeling of small or asymmetrical breasts as pathological conditions. Women, too, become involved in this process when they rely on plastic surgery as a solution for their problems. How do women participate in this medicalization process? How do predominating beliefs about medicine (as well as cultural assumptions about femininity) shape the decision to receive breast implants, and how do these beliefs and assumptions affect the ways in which women experience the outcomes of their surgeries?

Women's experiences with breast implants demonstrate how scientific and medical knowledge is uncertain, ambiguous, and continuously evolving. Since the development of breast implants in the early 1960s, medical scientists and epidemiologists have argued over whether the devices pose a serious threat to women's health. The media did not begin informing the public about this debate until the early 1990s, when the FDA was deciding whether or not to restrict the use of implants and when increasing numbers of women were alleging that they had been harmed by the devices. Since this time, numerous studies have been conducted to evaluate the risks associated with breast implants. While most of these studies conclude that the relationship between the devices and various diseases is "insignificant," anecdotal evidence continues to suggest otherwise. Consequently, many physicians and medical scientists are still unsure about how to interpret the scientific evidence regarding implant-related risk. If these "experts" are unable to come to an agreement about the risks associated with breast implants, how do implant recipients themselves make sense of the scientific "evidence"?

Moreover, how do these women respond to the medical uncertainty associated with a device that is intrinsically linked to their own feelings about themselves as "feminine"? Do women rely on the medical community for interpretation of the scientific evidence regarding implant-related risk? If not, where do they turn to make sense of the conflicting information? Finally, what do women perceive as the consequences of acknowledging a potential relationship between implants and disease? And how might coming to terms with these consequences relate to transformations in self, identity, and ideas about femininity and womanhood?

In the summer of 1993, I began placing announcements about my research in local newspapers and women's health newsletters, hoping to find women who had breast implants who were willing to let me interview them. I also located a support group for women with breast implants in the Boston area and, through a friend and professional colleague, found a plastic surgeon who said that he was willing to inform his patients with breast implants about my research.

Although I had these leads, by the end of the summer, I had conducted only three interviews with women. All of these women were members of the Boston support group. The group had over twenty members who had received breast implants. Nevertheless, their leader explained to me that women were hesitant to participate in my study because they did not feel comfortable sharing their personal experiences with a stranger. Many had not even told their own husbands that they had received breast implants. In addition, even though the plastic surgeon I had been in contact with had agreed to help me with recruitment, he never returned my phone calls. When I was finally able to reach him, he explained that he was no longer interested in my project. This was a typical response from most of the plastic surgeons I contacted.

In the fall of 1993, the American Society of Plastic and Reconstructive Surgeons responded to one of my announcements with a letter explaining that the society would be delighted to assist me with my research. About a week later, I contacted the society's media coordinator, who kindly provided me with a list of about ten plastic surgeons practicing in the Northeast. However, after making several calls, I found only one surgeon out of those listed who was interested in helping recruit women for my project. Although I was able to interview one of his patients, soon thereafter he, too, backed out of his commitment to assist me. In an apologetic tone, he explained that he had spoken with his lawyer, who thought he was "crazy" for becoming involved in a project that would only "stir up trouble" among implant recipients who might already be anxious about the recent media attention focusing on potential problems with the devices.

I found plastic surgeons' reluctance to assist me interesting and significant to my research. The ways in which they responded to my project demonstrated their unwillingness to acknowledge the possibility of a link between implants and disease and provided at least one possible explanation for this resistance—they were afraid of potential lawsuits. Nevertheless, I was disappointed, particularly since I was still having trouble finding women to interview. A year after I began my research, I had interviewed only about twenty women. Only two women had responded to my announcements in local papers. I had met a couple of them through family and friends, and others I found through attorneys' offices handling breast implant litigation. A Boston law firm was particularly helpful with providing me names of women who had received breast implants. All of these women were participating in a worldwide breast implant settlement arranged by lawyers and implant manufacturers to compensate women who alleged that they had been harmed by the devices.[6] A woman in Philadelphia (whom I call Tracy) who was involved with this settlement also helped me find respondents for my study. Tracy herself had received breast implants and was chosen by her law firm to be a contact person for other recipients of these devices. The firm was so inundated with calls from frightened women who had recently learned about the risks associated with their implants that it began referring many of them to Tracy, who was well informed about the medical and legal issues surrounding the devices. I had already contacted Tracy after finding her name on a list sent to me by a national support group for women with breast implants. Tracy not only gave me names of women to interview but also allowed me to interview her about her own implant-related experiences.

Throughout the spring and early summer of 1994, as I continued to read literature and news reports about breast implants, I came across the names of about fifty breast implant support groups and information networks. Most of the groups were located on the West Coast or other places far from my home; nevertheless, I wrote to all of them explaining the purpose of my research, hoping to find women to participate in my study. Since I knew from prior experience that many women felt that their implant-related experiences were "private matters," not to be shared with outsiders, I did not expect to receive many responses from women. To my surprise, however, I gradually began receiving phone calls, letters, and even personal essays about women's implant-related experiences from women all over the country—Colorado, Kansas, Idaho, Florida, Texas, New Jersey, New York, and even Alaska. Since I did not have the time or the resources to travel to all of these places, I decided to focus on California, the state from which I had received the largest cluster of responses.

In total, I conducted forty interviews with women who had received breast implants. Twenty-five of the women in my sample had breast implants for "cosmetic" reasons. According to popular belief, cosmetic surgery involving breast implants enhances the size and shape of women's breasts. However, only eleven of the twenty-five women who deemed their surgery "cosmetic" had received implants for this purpose. Twelve women had implants not to enlarge their breasts, but to lift their breast tissue after it had sagged following a pregnancy, nursing, or losing weight. Two of the twenty-five women had implants because their breasts were slightly asymmetrical.

Thirteen of the women I interviewed received breast implants for "reconstructive" purposes. Generally, breast reconstruction refers to the replacement of one or both breasts following a mastectomy. However, women who have severely asymmetrical breasts or congenital deformities of the breast also undergo "reconstructive" implant mammaplasty. Of the thirteen women I interviewed who had breast reconstruction, ten had implants following a mastectomy, one because her breasts were asymmetrical from a spinal deformity, one because her breast tissue decreased in volume after nursing, and one because she had "severely sagging" breasts.

Two of the forty women I interviewed were not sure how to respond to my question regarding the "type" of procedure they had. In other words, they were uncertain about whether their surgeries were deemed "reconstructive" or "cosmetic." One of these women stated that she sought implants because her breasts were "tubular," the other because her breasts were asymmetrical. One way to determine what type of procedure women had was to ask them whether insurance covered the cost of their surgeries. Third-party payers generally reimburse for surgeries deemed by physicians as "reconstructive," since they are perceived as "medically necessary." However, they do not reimburse for elective or

Table 1.1 Respondents who had "cosmetic" implant mammaplasty

Name of respondent	Date of surgery	Age at time of surgery
Christine	1970	29
Gayle	1971	29
Ann	1972	22
Barbara	1972	31
Lorraine	1972	29
Sheila	1973	29
Gwen	1974	30
Liz	1975	29
Mona	1975	28
Jane	1977	29
Karen	1977	18
Beth	1981	23
Joyce	1982	25
Nina	1983	27
Hillary	1986	38
Leslie	1986	20
Rose	1986	39
Gina	1987	33
Sophie	1988	28
Jenna	1989	32
Patty	1989	27
Alice	1990	34
Georgine	1990	32
Tracy	1990	43
Carmen	1992	21

Total = 25

"cosmetic" procedures. Insurance only partially covered both of the women's surgeries, leaving the question of "type" of procedure, in these two cases, unresolved.

At the time I conducted the interviews, the women ranged in age between twenty-three and seventy-two. Seven women had received breast implants before turning twenty-five; twenty more between the ages of twenty-five and thirty-five; nine more between thirty-five and forty-five; and three more between the ages of fifty and sixty-five. Of the forty women I spoke with, twenty-two were married, eight were divorced, three were separated and seven had never been married. All of the women who were divorced or separated had been married at the time they received breast implants. Thirty-six of the women I inter-

Table 1.2 Respondents who had "reconstructive" implant mammaplasty

Name of respondent	Date of surgery	Age at time of surgery
Grace	1971	19
Frances*	1975	32
Rita*	1978	42
Eleanor	1981	36
Paula*	1982	41
Suzanne*	1983	38
Abby*	1985	28
Brenda*	1986	43
Rebecca*	1986	39
Eve	1986	29
Mary*	1986	64
Maureen*	1987	53
Kate*	1989	64

Total = 13

*Women who had breast reconstruction after mastectomies

Table 1.3 Respondents who had implant mammaplasty for other reasons*

Name of respondent	Date of surgery	Age at time of surgery
Sarah	1980	20
Gloria	1983	39

Total = 2

*Sarah received implants because her breasts were "tubular," and Gloria received them because her breasts were "asymmetrical."

viewed identified themselves as white, one as Asian, two as Latino, and one as Native American. Seventeen women were employed, nine were homemakers, three were students, and eleven were currently unemployed. Of these eleven women, one reported that she was currently looking for a job; the remaining ten women stated that they had lost their jobs because they were too ill to work. These women were on disability insurance because they had been diagnosed with an illness that prevented them from participating in the workforce. Most of the women in my sample were well educated. Seven women had high school diplomas, twenty-three had attended either a two- or four-year college, and nine had advanced professional or master's degrees. One woman had completed a doctoral degree.

Twenty out of the forty women I interviewed had their breast implants removed because they experienced symptoms or complications associated with these devices. Complications included implant encapsulation that led to a severe hardening of the breasts, implant deflation, and ruptures. The symptoms women experienced ranged in severity from minor aching joints to debilitating pain and chronic fatigue. Other symptoms included hair loss, stomach irritability, rashes, fevers, and allergic reactions to certain foods and chemicals found in, for example, perfumes and household cleansers. Several women were diagnosed with atypical connective tissue diseases such as fibromyalgia and chronic fatigue syndrome. Others were diagnosed with classic forms of lupus, scleroderma, and Sjögren's syndrome. Not every woman who experienced implant-related symptoms had her implants removed. In total, thirty-four of the forty women I initially interviewed experienced physical symptoms or illnesses they suspected to be implant-related. Thirty-five women in the sample also reported having experienced complications directly related to their implants.

According to recent studies, my sample closely represents the larger population of one to two million women with breast implants in terms of race, class, marital status, and age. National averages compiled by the American Society of Plastic and Reconstructive Surgeons in 1990 show that 80 percent of all women receiving the most commonly performed cosmetic surgeries (including breast augmentation, liposuction, and collagen injections) are white.[7] Similarly, research conducted by Robert Cook and colleagues found that in 1989, implant mammaplasty was more common among white women than among minority groups.[8] This study also demonstrates that implant recipients tend to be of the higher socioeconomic classes and live in southern or western regions of the United States. Another study on trends in the utilization of silicone breast implants between 1964 and 1991 found that the majority of women receiving implants were married at the time of their surgeries and that there was a wide age variation among these implant recipients (between fifteen and seventy-nine years old).[9] The results of this study and other estimates[10] show that more women receive breast implants for cosmetic reasons than for reconstructive purposes (although the proportion of women receiving implants for breast cancer mastectomy reconstruction has increased over recent years[11]).

Although my study may be representative of the total population of women with breast implants in terms of various sociodemographic characteristics, it may be biased in other ways. For instance, I recruited the majority of my respondents from support groups and attorneys' offices handling breast implant litigation. These women were more likely to have experienced implant-related concerns, symptoms, and complications than women who were not members of support groups or pursuing legal action against implant manufacturers or plastic surgeons.[12] If I had been able to find more respondents through plastic surgeons' offices, the results of this study might have been different on several accounts. For instance, in order to protect their professional reputations, physicians might have referred me only to those patients who were pleased with the outcomes of their reconstructive or cosmetic surgeries. I speculate that these women would have been less willing to acknowledge a possible link between breast implants and disease and more likely to trust medical and scientific explanations about the risks and benefits associated with these devices. The majority of women I interviewed, on the other hand, had recognized the fallibility of medical science, enabling them to take a political, activist stance about their implant-related symptoms and concerns.

My recruitment strategy also influenced my own stance on the breast implant controversy. After listening to so many implant recipients talk about similar types of symptoms and implant-related complications, I came to believe that a link between silicone and disease exists. Yet, the intent of my research has never been to prove or disprove a relationship between breast implants and illness. No definitive conclusion about the risk of silicone can be based on a sample size of only forty women. Rather, my purpose is to demonstrate how women themselves participate in the medicalization of femininity by choosing to have breast implants, how they make sense of the medical and scientific uncertainty surrounding a controversial medical device, and how they, ironically, can become empowered by their illness experiences. In this way, I hope readers will view this book not as "evidence" supporting the dangers of silicone, but as a case study that sheds light on the process whereby beliefs about gender interact with prevailing expectations of medicine and science, shaping the structure and organization of medical care, as well as women's personal, daily life experiences.

Since the time of my last interview in 1994, new epidemiological evidence emerged suggesting that there is not a significant relationship between breast implants and disease. Marcia Angell, the executive editor of the *New England Journal of Medicine*, pursued this same conclusion in her 1996 book entitled *Science on Trial: The Clash of Medical Evidence and the Law in the Breast Implant Case.*[13] The book not only conveys the message that breast implants are "safe," but also condemns the Food and Drug Administration (FDA) for restricting the use of the devices, journalists for creating an atmosphere of alarm and fear among implant recipients, and, most of all, greedy plaintiff attorneys who, without scientific evidence, manipulated juries into having sympathy for women who alleged they were harmed by the devices. The book received widespread media attention and positive reviews in national newspapers and prestigious academic journals.[14] If implant recipients were aware of the most recent studies and publications concluding that breast implants pose no serious threat to women's health, I wanted to know how they were responding to them.

I conducted six follow-up interviews with women who expressed differing views about the breast implant controversy during my initial interviews with them. For instance, one of the six women who had her implants removed because she was fearful of developing disabling symptoms had started her own support network for women experiencing implant-related problems; whereas another woman who received an implant following a mastectomy had expressed to me her opinion that implants are "safe" and should still be made available to women. Over the past year, I discovered that many of the support groups and information networks for breast implant recipients have created home pages on the World Wide Web with links to message boards where women can discuss the latest publications regarding implants (including Angell's book) and find fact sheets about breast implant litigation and bibliographies listing the latest scientific and epidemiological studies on the risks associated with these devices.[15] Based on these discussions and my follow-up interviews, I found that the medical community's recent proclamation that implants are "safe" has reassured those women who remain satisfied with the outcomes of their breast surgeries, but has reinforced feelings of anger and disillusionment among those women who were already certain that their implants caused them harm.

A Meeting with Abby: Giving Women Voice

Although Abby resides in northern California, I scheduled a meeting with her while she was visiting her mother in southern Massachusetts—about thirty miles from my home in Providence, Rhode Island. Before I met Abby, I was driving all over Massachusetts, Connecticut, and

Pennsylvania visiting women who had agreed to let me interview them about their experiences with breast implants. I did not usually mind the long drives since they gave me plenty of time to reflect upon my research, but the thought of not having to travel far for an interview was also appealing. Although she appeared to be a young woman (maybe in her mid-thirties), Abby had a weathered look about her—her face was flushed and she looked tired and worn. Maybe it was just the summer heat and humidity. Although we had had only one phone conversation prior to our meeting, I felt surprisingly comfortable with Abby. My comfort with her may have been attributable to the fact that she had coordinated a support group of over four hundred implant recipients, making her an expert at talking and listening to women. Abby's friendly rapport with her mother, along with my meeting her in the home where she had grown up, may have clued me in as to the kind of person Abby was much sooner than if our first meeting had occurred somewhere else. I conducted most interviews with women in their own homes [16] and had witnessed many of their interactions with spouses and children, but the glimpse into Abby's past felt special.

Most people I talked to seemed to use the interview as an opportunity to piece together and make sense of their life histories with breast implants. Abby's replies to my questions did not reflect the same pattern of responses. Throughout our interview, Abby talked about the members of the support group she had organized in northern California. She did not go into specific details about individual members, but talked about their shared feelings and experiences. I realized that she had little desire to convey to me her own personal suffering as it related to her experiences with breast cancer, the subsequent loss of her breast, and her reconstructive surgery with a breast implant. Abby seemed to have no intention of discussing her own fear of medical uncertainty, nor did she wish to go into depth about the extent of her implant-related symptoms. In fact, Abby continually redirected her responses to my questions away from her own personal experiences with the implant she had received following her mastectomy to the common feelings and experiences shared by the members of her group. For instance, when I asked Abby if she had any problems or complications with her implant, she explained:

> I had a rupture, then I had the implant removed. The rupture caused silicone to spread all over. But, what we [support group members] found out through some research is that even if we don't have a rupture, the minute they put it in your body, it leaks out through the shell in molecules and goes all over—it

attacks the brain, lungs, heart, and liver. It goes for smooth muscles. A lot of us have only two-thirds lung capacity.

Similarly, when I asked her to describe her own implant-related symptoms she replied:

> Well, I have hot flashes—we [support group members] used to call them hot flashes but decided that a better term is "flushings." You get like so hot that you are burning from the inside. And, the women sometimes will actually have a burning sensation at the site of where the silicone has migrated—like you can feel the silicone in your body, in your chest or wherever. There are a lot of women who are getting breast cancer and they haven't been able to find the lumps because the implants get in the way of mammography. We believe some of the ladies in our group are getting cancer from their implants.

Finally, after I asked Abby to talk about her sexual and social life following the removal of her implant, she, again, responded by talking about the members of her group:

> Of course, I don't feel the same sexually. All of our sexual lives are not the same as they were before. I feel so badly. Myself—I can deal with what I look like now, but women whose breasts were fine—maybe they sagged, or they were small—for these women [removal] is such a traumatic thing. I have a lot of women in the group who are in their forties, thirties, and twenties. You know, once you start learning what the silicone is doing to your body you want to get it out. But, psychologically, you don't want to get it out because you know you are going to be maimed.

Abby was clearly on a mission to educate others by speaking out for all women who had received breast implants and experienced the same physical symptoms and feelings of embarrassment and shame that Abby herself experienced after she began suspecting that her implant was causing her problems. Abby was channeling women's collective feelings and experiences with implants through her own single voice.

Since Abby was a leader of a support group for women with breast implants, I asked her if she would mind informing members of her group about my research. Not only did Abby agree to assist me with recruitment, but she insisted that I make plans to stay with her while conducting my research in the San Francisco area. I was hesitant to take Abby up on her generous offer, but I agreed. Before I left, Abby held out her arms to give me a friendly embrace, saying, "You are part of our family now, Susan, a 'silicone sister.'" After my interview with Abby, my commitment toward my research took on a deeper sense of personal responsibility than it had in the past. Like Abby, I, too, wanted women's voices to be heard.

One month after our interview, I flew out to Los Angeles, where I conducted a handful of interviews, then drove up the coast and headed toward San Francisco. I stayed at Abby's home for about a week. During this time, Abby introduced me to the coleader of her group, Paula, and other group members. Even though I had rented a car and was fairly good at following directions, Abby insisted that she drive me to and from interviews. Most of the time she would go into another room where she would sit and collate newsletters or medical literature on breast implants to distribute to her group. However, on two visits, respondents asked me if Abby could remain present during our meeting. I initially thought this was not a good idea, worrying that women might not be as candid with Abby present. Nevertheless, I agreed to try it out and was reassured to find that Abby's presence seemed to comfort women rather than make them feel ill at ease. Moreover, Abby explained that she never had the opportunity to listen to women tell their implant-related stories from beginning to end and found that listening to the interviews gave her deeper insights into the extent of some women's emotional and physical suffering.

The interviews were very much a two-way street. I was taping the women's accounts of their experiences with breast implants, but many women wanted to know what kind of person I was, whether I was married or involved in a relationship, and how I became interested in this research. Some asked if I had breast implants. Other questions focused on information seeking. For instance, some women who were not members of support groups wanted to join one, asking me if I knew of any nearby. Women also wanted to know if other women I had interviewed were experiencing implant-related symptoms or complications. Another group of questions women posed to me centered around their seeking validation and reassurance for their troubles and concerns. Women who were sick and believed their symptoms were linked to their implants wanted to know if I thought they were "crazy" for thinking this. Similarly, one woman I interviewed wanted to know if I thought her decision to receive implants seemed "irrational."

Another researcher, Ann Oakley, was faced with similar types of questions from women she interviewed during her research on motherhood.[17] Oakley had turned to methodology textbooks for advice. These books warn interviewers of the dangers associated with respondents' questions, suggesting strategies of avoidance. For example, one book recommended laughing off respondents' questions in order to avoid revealing personal opinions—behaving otherwise might "bias" the interview. Oakley argues, however, that when interviewing women about a sensitive issue "an attitude of refusing to answer questions or offer any kind of personal feedback [is] not helpful in terms of the traditional goal of promoting 'rapport.'"[18] Deciding to depart from conventional interviewing ethics, she answered her respondents' questions honestly and openly. In fact, Oakley progressively moved away from perceiving her respondents as simply passive informants, to viewing them as co-investigators.

During the course of my own research I, too, found that I was able to establish women's trust when I responded truthfully to their questions. I shared with them information about my personal life; told them that, no, I did not have breast implants; was honest when they asked me questions about other women's implant-related experiences; and when they asked, I provided them with information about breast implant support groups and information networks. I also tried to validate women's experiences. When women asked me if I felt that their problems were "all in their heads," I said no, telling them that I had visited many other women who described implant-related symptoms and complications similar to their own. When I could see that women were having a difficult time talking about their experiences with breast implants—if their eyes began to water or if they broke down in tears—I would reassure them that they were not alone.

Women shared intimate details of their lives.[19] They told me about their views on sexuality and intimacy, relating these issues to their perceptions of their own bodies, as well as their relationships with spouses and lovers. Some talked about the sense of inner conflict they experienced about having undergone plastic surgery. Although some women were glad to have received implants and were happy with their new bodies, others felt guilty about enlarging or reconstructing their breasts. These women regretted having taken such a drastic step to feel more "feminine" or more "like a woman." Many women conveyed to me feelings of self-blame and guilt after learning about the potential risks associated with breast implants. How could they have agreed to allow someone insert a "dangerous" substance into their healthy bodies, simply for the sake of improving their appearances? More frequently, however, women expressed to me their anger as they directed blame at the medical community for not taking their implant-related complaints seriously and the government for not taking a more active role in recognizing the extent of anxiety, confusion, and harm that breast implants had caused women. Women also shared with me the depth of their fears and anxieties about the uncertainty of their futures. Many talked about the physical symptoms they began experiencing after receiving breast implants and wondered if their worsening health was connected to these devices. In short, my transcripts of these interviews provided me with deeply moving personal accounts of women's most intimate feelings about health and illness, their sexual and social lives, and their sense of who they were in relation to the physical appearance of their bodies.

2

Historical Background
The Emergence of a Controversy

*F*or decades, women have enhanced the size and shape of their breasts using a variety of methods, including exercises, creams, and padded or push-up bras. Over the past fifty years, American women also have turned to plastic surgery to meet society's ideal. Since the post–World War II era, physicians have used liquid silicone injections and implantable devices to enlarge women's breasts. While some of these procedures are now prohibited from use because they are believed to cause a variety of health problems and complications among women, the insertion of breast implants into women's bodies has remained a popular way of increasing female breast size for over thirty years. Between one and two million women have received breast implants.[1] Prior to 1992, approximately 150,000 women received implants annually—20 percent for reconstructive purposes following mastectomies and 80 percent for cosmetic reasons to enlarge healthy breasts.[2] One estimate suggests that since 1994, close to 70,000 women a year continue to undergo this surgery.[3] Implant mammaplasty to enlarge women's breasts is a relatively simple surgical procedure. Most of the women I interviewed explained that the actual surgery lasted only about an hour and that they were able to return home the same day the procedure was performed. Cosmetic surgery involving breast implants requires only a small incision underneath the breast in order to insert the soft, pliable implant. For better cosmetic results, some surgeons insert implants through the nipple, and more recently, a few have tried inserting them via the navel.[4]

In the early 1950s, some physicians implanted women's bodies with prosthetic sponges to enhance their breast size. Plastic surgeons discontinued this practice after learning that the procedure resulted in many serious postoperative complications. In particular, fatty tissue would grow into the devices, causing women's breasts to become extremely hard and painful. Injecting women's breasts with liquid silicone and the insertion of breast implants into women's bodies also have a long history of serious side effects. Nevertheless, physicians continued to perform these procedures, despite their knowledge of the risks associated with them. Plastic surgeons' establishment of a psychiatric justification for breast augmentation, along with the heightened public awareness of surgical breast enhancement in the 1960s, led to the widespread use of silicone breast injections. Although this procedure was eventually prohibited, the reasons behind its popularity paved the way for the development and extensive use of silicone breast implants throughout the 1970s and 1980s.

Since the early 1960s, when the first breast implant was created, the device has been associated with a number of complications, such as infections, ruptures, and hardening of the breasts. By the late 1980s, medical literature also began reporting on various systemic reactions and autoimmune illnesses related to breast implants. The media's dissemination of this information has fueled a scientific and public debate over whether or not breast implants are safe, leading the Food and Drug Administration (FDA) to restrict the use of silicone breast implants in 1992. Since then, the breast implant controversy has left women who have implants anxious and frightened about the uncertainty of their futures, and plastic surgeons fearful of losing what has become for them a $3 million business.[5]

Since the 1960s, medical scientists have never claimed that breast implants (or any other procedure to enlarge women's breasts) are entirely risk-free. Nevertheless, most plastic surgeons have continued to recommend these devices to their female patients. Even though scientists have yet to determine whether breast implants pose a serious threat to women's health, the overall conclusion that plastic surgeons have drawn is that their benefits (that is, providing women with larger, more shapely breasts) far outweigh any "possible" risks.

Discovering Applications for Silicone

In the early 1940s, Dow Corning Corporation developed the synthetic compound silicone. Derived from sand and quartz, silicone was perceived by scientists as possessing remarkable qualities: It did not react with most chemicals, was stronger than plastic and more flexible than glass, and could withstand amazingly high temperatures—up to 900 degrees Fahrenheit. Moreover, scientists could change the consistency of silicone from a solid to a fluid state, depending on temperature and pressure. With these properties, Dow Corning was able to find a wide range of applications for its new substance. First used as a sealant for ignition systems on World War II aircraft, by the early 1950s, silicone became widely used for many different industrial and household purposes. For instance, a liquid form of the substance was developed to lubricate high-performance machinery, to waterproof leather, and to clean optical equipment. A semisolid form of silicone was created to caulk bathtubs and seal cracks in walls. Silicone also was transformed into a rubberlike substance to create infant pacifiers. Yet another application of the compound resulted in the development of Silly Putty, the soft, pliable, gooey substance sold in a plastic egg to children as a toy since the 1960s.[6]

By the 1960s, researchers and scientists began to discover medical applications for silicone. Physicians began coating needles with liquid silicone to facilitate delivery of injections into the body. The compound was transformed into tubing for blood and dialysis equipment, and prostheses for joints and cartilage replacements. The ability of silicone to transform from a solid to liquid state led researchers to believe that it could also be used in the field of plastic surgery: "Even highly viscous silicone oils that were nearly completely 'gelled' would be fluid enough to be injected when put under the pressure of a hypodermic needle. Once injected into the body, such oils would be expected to assume a quasi-solid consistency at body temperature and yet stay in place where injected because of the coherence of the gel."[7]

With this characteristic, plastic surgeons could inject liquid silicone into human bodies. Believing the substance was biologically inert and an "ideal soft-tissue substitute," they used it to fill in soft-tissue facial defects and to smooth out wrinkled skin. They also began to inject liquid silicone directly into women's breasts to make them larger.[8]

Breast Injections, the Prosthetic Sponge, and a Medical Justification for Breast Enhancement

Even though silicone was created in the United States, its use in breast injections did not originate here. That application began in Japan shortly after World War II, when American forces still occupied that country. Because American servicemen had a reputation for preferring women with breasts larger than those of most Japanese women, Japanese cosmetologists began experimenting with various substances and procedures to enlarge the breasts of Japanese prostitutes. Initially, this was accomplished by directly injecting substances such as goats' milk and mixtures of paraffin and petroleum jelly into women's breasts.[9] Later, cosmetologists began to perform the procedure using liquid silicone. Migration of the liquid could be prevented by adding olive or cottonseed oil, which would cause immediate scarring and thus encapsulate the silicone at the site of injection.[10] Dr. Sakurai was the first to use silicone injections in Japan and, shortly thereafter, introduced his technique to the United States, opening up a practice in California, where breast injections (later to be known as "Sakurai formula") became especially popular. By 1965, more than seventy-five plastic surgeons in Los Angeles alone were injecting women's breasts with silicone.[11]

While Sakurai had familiarized the medical community with silicone injections, Carol Doda was probably the individual who introduced the general public to this procedure. Doda was a topless dancer at the Condor Club in San Francisco in the 1960s; she attracted widespread media attention after she had her own breasts enhanced with silicone injections. Immediately, she went from "a rather ordinary go-go dancer with a 36-inch bust to a 44-inch topless superstar."[12] Subsequently, the practice of breast injections became popular in other states such as Nevada and Texas where nightclubs commonly used topless dancing and hired busty women to lure in customers. An estimated fifty thousand American women have had their breasts injected with liquid silicone since the late 1940s, when the procedure was first introduced to the United States.[13]

Even though silicone was believed to be a biologically inert and non-reactive substance, women who had undergone breast injections experienced many serious complications. For instance, some experienced ulceration, scarring, and swelling around their breasts. Others suffered from gangrene, infections, and collapsed lungs. Yet another problem resulted from the migration of silicone to various parts of women's bodies. Although injections were often altered with oil that was intended to cause scarring to prevent migration, masses of silicone occasionally made their way to other parts of women's bodies. Sometimes these masses could be surgically removed successfully. However, more frequently, physicians were unable to excise the large quantities of the gel without disfiguring women. At least four deaths have been attributed to silicone injections. In one of these cases, silicone had migrated to a woman's lungs, causing her to suffocate.[14]

Prior to the widespread use of silicone injections in the United States, some physicians used implantable sponges as a soft-tissue substitute. Made from polyvinyl alcohol (Ivalon), the implantable sponge was created by Doctors J. H. Grindlay and D. T. Clagette in 1949. These medical scientists believed they had developed an ideal prosthetic material that could be used for many surgical purposes, such as filling out soft-tissue defects and replacing areas of cartilage and bone loss.[15] The sponge was also used extensively for augmentation mammaplasty.[16] However, the use of the device for this purpose was short-lived. Since the sponge had no outer envelope to prevent human tissue from growing into it, scar tissue frequently developed around the implant, squeezing women's breasts into very tight, hard balls. Many women reported that their breasts became painful and that their breast size eventually decreased after the surgical procedure. In one study the volume of sponges decreased by 20 to 50 percent.[17] An earlier report suggested that Ivalon was carcinogenic in rodents.[18]

The risks involved with the Ivalon sponge led some researchers to believe that liquid silicone was the ideal soft-tissue substitute. Aware of problems associated with the silicones injected by Japanese cosmetologists and physicians, Herbert Conway and Dicran Goulian conducted a study on "injectable silastic RTV," a newer, improved, "jellylike" silicone formula.[19] In their preliminary report of the substance, these researchers concluded:

> Although the results following use of this jellylike silicone leave something to be desired, some of the major disadvantages of the sponge type of implants are not encountered. . . . The risk of serious complications resulting from infection is significantly reduced. . . . Although this material in its final pros-

thetic form is more dense than the surrounding soft tissues, this variation is not significant. Moreover, the jellylike silicone does not increase in hardness with the passage of time as do the implants of sponge.[20]

Conway and Goulian experimented on a number of human subjects, injecting silicone into their bodies for a variety of problems, including facial hemiatrophy, posttraumatic molar deformity, and "micromastia" —the medical term that was increasingly used among physicians to refer to "small breasts." The researchers reported that the only complication in their experiment occurred after they injected a woman's breasts with the substance: "The mixture did not set evenly. The breast had such an irregular appearance that the prosthesis was removed."[21] Some physicians believed that the risks associated with inserting sponges into women's breasts were far greater than an irregular appearance; the sponges were so porous that soft tissue inevitably grew into them, causing "capsular contracture," a term used to describe the formation of scar tissue around the devices. This complication often resulted in a painful hardening of women's breasts.

Even though the use of the implantable sponge was short-lived, it paved the way for the establishment of what the medical community perceived as a legitimate reason for providing women with larger breasts. According to plastic surgeons, augmentation mammaplasty improved women's "self-esteem," providing them with an entirely new emotional outlook. One of the earliest studies on the psychiatric implications of breast enhancement on women was conducted in 1958, by M. T. Edgerton and A. R. McClary.[22] These researchers claimed that the thirty-two women who participated in their study on augmentation mammaplasty with the Ivalon sponge were all diagnosed as "emotionally ill" prior to their surgeries: "All patients psychiatrically studied, were noted to be involved in major life adjustment situations, usually separation and divorce. The common denominator was an unrecognized depressive reaction which was disguised beneath their fixations of feelings upon their breasts. . . . The small size of the breasts demonstrated to the world that they lacked something—were empty."[23]

Edgerton and McClary's depiction of the women they studied is infused with Freudian, psychoanalytic language. According to the researchers, the feeling of "emptiness" the women experienced was primarily rooted in their relationships with their fathers. Women who wanted to have their breasts surgically enhanced felt that having small breasts was "a kind of punishment." Edgerton and McClary attributed the deepest meaning of this punishment to women's guilt about affectionate and sexual feelings for their fathers. For these women, breasts symbolized a "measure of [their] father's love—'that something a girl should get from her father.'"[24] Thus, the "therapeutic" nature of receiving implants was linked to the "unique structuring of the surgeon-patient relationship." Women who underwent the procedure experienced a "miraculous change in inner feelings because that something that [they] had needed for so long had been given to [them] (by the surgeon?)."[25]

In short, Edgerton and McClary believed that female patients who desire larger breasts are secretly in love with their fathers who never gave them enough attention while growing up. Surgeons can serve as the male, fatherlike figure to these emotionally tormented women, offering them that love and tenderness (as symbolized by the breast) that their own fathers never gave them. This explanation for why women seek breast enhancement clearly epitomizes the asymmetrical and sexist nature of the relationship between the powerful, all-knowing, male physician and the passive, emotionally distraught, female patient. Nevertheless, it reflected a growing trend within the field of plastic surgery.

As early as the 1930s, Freudian language appeared elsewhere in the medical literature on cosmetic surgery. Plastic surgeons viewed their patients' desires to reshape or alter various parts of their bodies in terms of displacement of deeper underlying conflicts. For instance, in an article published in 1934, Howard Updegraff and Karl Menninger described one case study of an adolescent boy who complained to a plastic surgeon about the size of his hands, which he felt appeared "too feminine."[26] The authors believed that the boy's complaint stemmed from his guilt associated with excessive masturbation. The patient felt emasculated not simply because his hands were too small, but because his genitals were too small—subconsciously, he believed that masturbation "had made him feminine."[27]

Hay's literature review on the psychiatric aspects of cosmetic rhinoplasty[28] provides further examples illustrating how Freudian language was used to justify plastic surgeons' practices. The review includes a case study of a man who turned to cosmetic surgery to resolve underlying psychological conflicts about his homosexual practices.[29] Unable to adjust or accept the "normal" male role, the patient opted to reshape his nose, unconsciously desiring a more "feminine" profile. Hay's review also includes a summary of a study[30] arguing that women who seek cosmetic rhinoplasty generally have poor relationships with mothers who served as poor identification models throughout their childhood. Identifying solely with their fathers led these women to develop psychosexual difficulties in later life. They subconsciously believed that they could resolve the problem of conflicted identification by reshaping their noses, which represented a paternal feature (i.e., the phallus).

Three years after the Edgerton and McClary study, Edgerton, E. Meyer, and W. E. Jacobson published further research that evaluated the psychiatric benefits of breast enhancement surgery with synthetic sponges.[31] The authors concluded that women's self-esteem improved and their sense of breast-consciousness was minimized following their operations. Moreover, the researchers stated that both women and their husbands "spoke with enthusiasm of improvement in marital happiness following the operation."[32] Even though plastic surgeons today define good candidates for breast enhancement as women who undergo the surgery "for themselves,"[33] in the 1950s, they commonly performed the operation on women who were experiencing marital problems and felt they could improve their relationships with their spouses (and, thus, improve their own "self-esteem") by enlarging their breasts. Although physicians stopped using the sponge soon after they discovered that women's breasts hardened and became painful after the procedure, some physicians did not follow the same course of action after they had learned about the dangers associated with silicone injections. By the 1960s, when breast injections were in widespread use, the psychiatric justification for augmentation mammaplasty had already been established. Moreover, breast injections in the mid-1960s began to receive widespread publicity with the claims of Carol Doda and other showgirls that "any girl can be as large as her dreams."[34] This public awareness of the procedure led to an increased demand for breast enhancement among the female population and provided plastic surgeons with a quick and simple way to make a profit. On average, plastic surgeons in the 1960s earned a thousand dollars every time they injected a woman's breasts with silicone.[35]

Both silicone breast injections and implantable sponges were used prior to federal regulations requiring proof of safety and effectiveness of medical devices. By the mid-1960s, the Food and Drug Administration (FDA) defined silicone as a "drug" and so began to regulate its use.[36] Physicians continued to use the substance for years following.

Dow Corning Corporation was still permitted to sell the compound to doctors who claimed they were conducting research on silicone, or who stated they were using the substance for approved uses—for example, as a lubricant for artificial joints and catheters. Although physicians were required to sign affidavits stating that they would not inject silicone into human beings, this did not prevent some of them from falsifying these documents, or even "buying industrial grade silicone in a hardware store, attempting to sterilize it, and then injecting it into women." [37] In Las Vegas, so many women had turned to physicians with problems resulting from silicone injections that the state of Nevada enacted emergency legislation in 1975 outlawing the procedure. California passed similar legislation the following year.

The Development of the Silicone Breast Implant

In search of a breast prosthesis that would produce a good cosmetic result and pose no threat to a woman's health, Doctors Frank Gerow and Thomas Cronin came up with the idea of encasing salt water inside a thin envelope of silicone polymer. However, Dow Corning's public relations representative, Silas Braley, convinced the doctors that filling the bag with a silicone gel would "duplicate the feeling of the normal breast." [38] Both Gerow and Cronin were aware of the problems associated with liquid silicone injections, but believed that if silicone gel was encased inside a thin envelope of silicone polymer, the substance would not migrate into women's bodies and cause complications. This assumption was not based on clinical trials involving human subjects, nor on animal studies. At the time, the FDA had no protocol for testing medical devices, nor did the administration have the jurisdiction to regulate these devices once they were in use. Since silicone had been employed in other medical applications, such as brain shunts for hydrocephalic children and bands around the eyeball for retinal detachments, without any reported complications or problems, Cronin and Gerow assumed that human bodies could tolerate a breast implant made of the substance. The researchers designed their first silicone breast prosthesis in 1961. In 1962, for the first time, the device was surgically implanted into a woman's body. [39]

In 1963, Cronin introduced the implant to the International Society of Plastic Surgeons, claiming that silicone was a totally inert substance. Since silicone had been used to create other medical devices with no evidence of serious risks, plastic surgeons were excited by the innovation and saw no reason to believe that it could be harmful to women. Soon thereafter, Cronin patented the implant as the "Cronin implant" and assigned the rights to Dow Corning Corporation. Although researchers never conducted formal clinical trials and safety testing of the device, the original patent describes it as being a "totally implantable, non-reactive device to be implanted within the human body."[40] By the mid-1960s, the Cronin breast implant was promoted and marketed with claims that the prosthesis was safe and approximated the "softness, contour, and fluid-like mobility of the normal breast."[41] Consequently, many plastic surgeons felt that these benefits far outweighed the minor risks associated with surgery. Finding no reason to doubt the safety of the prosthesis, they assumed it would remain intact within a woman's body over her entire lifetime.

In reality, the early versions of the implant were fraught with serious complications. In order to secure the implant to the pectoral muscle, posterior Dacron patches were attached to the rear of the prosthesis. The patches sometimes induced an intense inflammatory reaction that often resulted in the formation of scar tissue around the device. This made implant removal, if problems arose, an "insurmountable surgical problem."[42] Ruptures and capsule formation around the prosthesis were further problems associated with these early implants. These complications led scientists, throughout the 1970s, to make many modifications on the devices in order to improve their effectiveness.

The Emergence and Government Regulation of Different Types of Implants[43]

Because breast implants were not regulated by the FDA in the early 1970s, manufacturers were free to develop variations of the original breast implant with few studies to demonstrate their safety and efficacy. Different implant manufacturers experimented with textured and smooth surfaces, as well as round and contour shapes, and used different materials both around and within implants to see what produced the best "cosmetic result." As a consequence, manufacturers achieved desirable results often at the expense of controlling the quality and safety of their products. Two examples of this negligence are the development and marketing of the polyurethane-foam-covered silicone implant, and, in the 1970s, the silicone-gel-filled breast implant. In each case, manufacturers had attempted to improve the "effectiveness" of breast implants, which often referred to how "natural" the devices appeared after they were implanted in women's bodies. Competing with other companies to produce an implant that gave the best cosmetic result, implant manufacturers paid little attention to problems associated with these devices. Consequently, the FDA has restricted the use of all silicone breast implants because manufacturers failed to provide evidence demonstrating their safety. To date, saline breast implants are the only implants available to women who wish them for either cosmetic purposes or reconstruction after breast cancer.

Saline Breast Implants

Saline implants were developed in the mid-1960s and are currently marketed as a safe alternative to the silicone-filled prosthesis. The saline implant is lined with a silicone envelope that, while empty, is surgically inserted into a woman's body and then filled with salt water through an exterior valve. Although reports indicate that ruptures and deflation are more common with saline implants than silicone devices, many researchers believe that they are safer than any other internal breast prosthesis since the saline resembles natural bodily fluid and can easily be absorbed without harm if the device happens to leak or break. Despite this knowledge, many plastic surgeons have opted not to use saline implants because they do not always produce the most "natural feel," or provide women with the best possible appearance.

While saline implants may be the safest internal breast prosthesis, evidence suggests that this implant has serious risks. For instance, women's bodies may react to the silicone envelope surrounding the implant, which can degrade shedding silicone particles into their bodies. Further evidence suggests that saline implants are more susceptible to rupture and rapid deflation, requiring further surgery. In addition to these problems, physicians since 1983 have concluded that in some cases saline can provide a medium for the growth of harmful bacteria.[44] On January 5, 1993, the FDA required manufacturers of saline breast implants to submit evidence of their safety and efficacy if they want to keep the devices on the market.[45] The FDA has yet to determine whether these devices pose a threat to women's health.

Polyurethane-Foam-Covered Implants

In the early 1970s, Heyer-Schulte Corporation, a California-based manufacturer, produced and marketed the polyurethane-foam-covered implant. In theory, the outer layer of foam prevents the formation of fibrous tissue growth around the breast implant (capsular contracture). This condition, which frequently leads to a painful hardening or distortion of the shape of the breast, is a common occurrence among women who have breast implants.[46] By the mid-1970s, Heyer-Schulte stopped producing the polyurethane-foam-covered implants due to growing concerns that the devices caused an inflammatory response among women who received them. Despite this warning, Aesthech Corporation (which was later bought out by Surgitek, a subsidiary of Bristol-Myers Squibb) took over the production and marketing of the foam-covered implants. By the late 1980s, these devices became the most popular breast implants on the market. Prior to 1990, between 200,000 and 400,000 women received the polyurethane-foam-covered prosthesis.[47]

Manufacturers of the polyurethane implants described the outer layer of foam as a "patented Microthane interface system."[48] A more common name for the material is "Scott Industrial Foam"—the same material that is used in furniture upholstery, carpet-cleaning equipment, and automobile air filters. In 1987, a Florida liability lawsuit was brought against manufacturers of these implants. During this case, the scientist who analyzed the polyurethane foam covering found that it contained traces of 2,4-toluene diamine (TDA), a substance that has been classified by the U.S. government as a hazardous waste and is a suspected human carcinogen. Not until the 1987 suit did officials from Scottfoam Industrial Corporation discover that their material was being implanted into human bodies.[49] Shocked by the news, the company's product control manager warned that the material was not meant for medical use and recommended that Aesthech discontinue implanting it into women's bodies. Nevertheless, the polyurethane foam surrounding the prosthesis diminished the risk of hardening and, thus, produced a good cosmetic result. Consequently, manufacturers continued to produce and distribute the implants, as profits from the device soared.

By the early 1990s, further studies confirmed that the polyurethane foam around implants can degrade into TDA,[50] and traces of the potential carcinogen were found in the urine and breast milk of women who had received the device.[51] Increasingly, women who had received these devices were filing lawsuits against implant manufacturers, alleging that they developed cancer and other diseases resulting from their exposure to polyurethane.

In 1990, the FDA finally began to investigate problems associated with the polyurethane-coated implants and, by April 1991, required Bristol-Myers Squibb to conduct postmarket surveillance on the risks of their product. In order to avoid further investigation, the company voluntarily withdrew the devices from the market in September 1991.

The 1970s Reformulation of the Silicone Implant

Presently, the most controversial implant is the silicone-gel-filled prosthesis that was first marketed in the early 1970s. During this time, Dow Corning and many other manufacturers moved to reformulate the original breast implant by changing the characteristics of both the outer envelope and the silicone gel held within it. The outer shell was made thinner, and the silicone gel was altered to a less viscous, fluid state in order to improve the natural feel of the breast implant, and thus lead to a better cosmetic result. Moreover, the new implants were so pliable that surgeons could insert them inside women's bodies through very small incisions that left unnoticeable scarring. Researchers now believe that these modifications are what prompted an increase in the documented cases of health problems and complications associated with breast implants.[52]

Beginning in 1978, evidence in medical journals increasingly suggested that the envelope of the breast implants created in the early 1970s was permeable. This meant that free-flowing silicone gel could slowly leak into women's bodies.[53] Apparently, the slow-leaking gel from the implant is evident to anybody who has held the prosthesis or placed the device on a piece of paper to witness the formation of a greasy stain.

Internal company memoranda revealed that Dow officials were fully aware that these new implants leaked before they marketed these devices. This evidence, consisting of internal memoranda and ninety scientific studies, had been sealed under a protective court order that Dow Corning obtained after settling a 1984 lawsuit brought by Maria Stern, the first woman to allege that her implants were linked to debilitating autoimmune symptoms and diseases. In this case, the jury concluded not only that Stern's illnesses were attributable to silicone, but found Dow Corning guilty of fraud. Dow appealed the case and lost, then appealed again. The case was settled out of court before the final ruling could be reached. Not only were Dow documents sealed after this ruling, but expert witnesses who appeared in the trial were sworn to secrecy about the case.[54]

Nevertheless, Sidney Wolfe, the director of Public Citizen Research Group, a nonprofit consumer advocacy group in Washington D.C., obtained one of the Dow documents—a study that concluded that silicone gel had caused cancer in over 23 percent of the laboratory animals in the research.[55] Wolfe held a news conference to report the study, then filed suit against the FDA, alleging that the agency was withholding important information from the public. The pending suit pressured the FDA to release Dow Corning company documents so that doctors and implant recipients would be aware of the risks associated with the devices. The studies and memoranda were made public on January 22, 1992.[56]

Among the public documents were letters written by Tom Talcott, a scientist at Dow Corning who consistently warned his colleagues at Dow about implant-related complications. For instance, in one letter, Talcott reported that sales representatives were complaining that the new implants leaked profusely.[57] Not only did manufacturers ignore Talcott's concern, but they also encouraged sales representatives to conceal the leak problem from plastic surgeons. One memo, written by a marketing executive at Dow to a sales representative, reads:

> It has been observed that the new [implants] . . . have a tendency to appear oily after being manipulated. This could prove to be a problem with your daily [sales presentations to doctors] where [implant] manipulation is a must. . . . Keep in mind that this is not a product problem; our technical people assure us that the doctor in the O.R. will not see any appreciable oiling on products removed from the package. The oily phenomenon seems to appear the day following manipulation. . . . You should make plans to change demonstration samples often. Also, be sure samples are clean and dry before customer detailing. Two easy ways to clean demonstration samples while traveling, 1) wash with soap and water in the nearest washroom, dry with hand towels. 2) Carry a small bottle of [cleaning fluid] and rag.[58]

Increasingly, evidence was surfacing that indicated that the new implants not only leaked but also were more susceptible to ruptures. In another memo, Talcott reported to his colleagues that two implants broke during augmentation surgery for a television tape demonstration.[59] Even Dr. Cronin, who had designed the original breast implant, reported that in one of his patients a straw-colored fluid oozed out of her breasts daily for one month. Upon removal of the implant, it was found that the device had ruptured.[60]

In the late 1970s, the medical literature began reporting pathological reactions to silicone from leaking and ruptured implants. For instance, one case study[61] reported that a woman nearly died after developing a number of systemic problems, including high fever, arthritis, and kidney failure following the leakage of silicone from her implant. Her health improved dramatically after her implants were removed.

Although Dow Corning and other manufacturers were aware that silicone-gel-filled breast implants could cause dangerous complications and harmful side effects, they continued to market the devices. Dow documents suggest that in order for the company to vie for a market share in what was becoming an increasingly competitive implant market, the manufacturers gave little attention to safety studies and looked the other way when problems with the device arose. Another of Talcott's memos to Dow executives states: "During our task force assignment to get the new products to market, a large number of people spent a lot of time discussing the envelope quality. We ended up saying the envelopes were 'good enough' while looking at gross thin spots and flaws in the form of significant bubbles."[62]

Throughout the 1980s and early 1990s increasing numbers of women began to experience problems associated with their silicone breast implants and voiced their concerns to the FDA. By December 1990, the FDA had received over four thousand reports of malfunctions or serious injury. This number was believed to represent only a small portion of the problems associated with the prosthesis since only about 5 percent of adverse effects of all medical devices and drugs are reported to the FDA.[63]

The FDA was aware of possible problems with implants since the 1970s, yet they did not have the authority to regulate the devices until 1976. In this year, the Medical Device Amendments to the Food, Drug and Cosmetic Act was passed, enabling the FDA to regulate medical devices after categorizing them into one of three classes, depending of their level of risk. Only the highest classification (Class III) would require manufacturers to provide evidence of a device's safety and efficacy before its marketing. The FDA was required to go back and request manufacturers to provide proof of the safety and effectiveness of medical devices already on the market, only if there was reason to do so. Because implant manufacturers and plastic surgeons claimed that breast implants had been on the market for over a decade without any evidence of medical risk or complications they (like many other medical devices) were "grandfathered" under the new law.[64]

By 1978, after concerned physicians and scientists complained to the FDA that implants leak and rupture,[65] an FDA advisory panel met to discuss the safety of the devices. Many of the plastic surgeons on the panel proposed classifying implants as Class II medical devices—a classification that would not require manufacturers to provide proof of safety and efficacy. Despite their recommendation, in 1983, the panel decided that all breast implants should be categorized as Class III devices. In June 1988, the classification was made official.[66] This meant that the FDA could require implant manufacturers "to submit premarket approval (PMA) applications for all breast implants, which would demonstrate safety and effectiveness."[67] Not until 1991 did the FDA demand that all manufacturers of breast implants submit PMA applications in order to review the safety and efficacy of the devices. The review process began in November 1991 in the form of public hearings before an FDA advisory panel. In December of this same year, Mariann Hopkins, a woman who had received breast implants following a bilateral mastectomy, won a $7.3 million lawsuit against Dow Corning Corporation. Hopkins filed her suit against the company in 1988, alleging that her implants caused her to develop mixed connective tissue disease and other serious health problems. Although Dow attempted to settle the case out of court, Hopkins turned down the company's monetary offers. She was determined to make the public aware of the health effects associated with breast implants and felt that if she accepted a settlement, the evidence about the risks associated with breast implants would remain sealed under protective court orders.[68]

Shortly after this case, on January 6, 1992, David Kessler, the commissioner of the FDA, declared a voluntary moratorium on the use of silicone gel breast implants because implant manufacturers failed to provide sufficient evidence proving the safety and efficacy of the devices, and increasing numbers of women were reporting problems. On April 16, 1992, the FDA announced that silicone breast implants would be available only through controlled, clinical trials and would be limited to women who wish them exclusively for either reconstructive purposes or for replacement of a ruptured implant. These women now fall under an "urgent need" classification.[69]

In the early 1990s, news reports and television shows increasingly disseminated information to the public about the possible dangers associated with leaking and ruptured implants. For instance, *Face to Face with Connie Chung* aired a show on December 10, 1990, which specifically called into question the risks associated with the polyurethane-covered silicone devices. In addition, talk show host Jenny Jones came forward about her own problems with silicone breast implants on her show that aired on October 12, 1992. Newspapers increasingly reported on implant-related risk, providing details to the public about manufacturer cover-ups and anecdotes from women who claimed they were harmed by the devices.[70] Moreover, in the early 1990s, implant recipients began to organize support groups for frightened and concerned women who wanted to learn about implant-associated risks, implant removal, treatments for implant-related symptoms and breast implant litigation.

By June 1992, the heightened public awareness of potential problems with breast implants resulted in a total of 14,259 reports to the FDA from women alleging they had experienced adverse reactions to these implants.[71] By the end of 1993, more than 12,000 women had filed lawsuits against Dow Corning Corporation claiming that the devices had harmed them.[72] The number of lawsuits brought against Dow and other implant manufacturers resulted in a $4.3 billion global settlement that was intended to offer compensation to any woman with diseases or symptoms allegedly associated with breast implants. The agreement was approved by implant manufacturers in March 1994;[73] however, since over 400,000 women filed claims under the settlement, the United States District Court Judge Sam C. Pointer Jr. declared that it was underfunded by at least $3 billion. Moreover, nearly 20,000 women opted to pursue individual lawsuits against implant manufacturers outside of the settlement. By July 1995, juries had awarded breast implant plaintiffs over $80 million in damages. This was the aftermath of only eleven trials—most of these cases were against the largest implant manufacturer, Dow Corning Corporation.[74] These events led Dow Corning to file for bankruptcy in 1995, freezing breast implant litigation against the company, and leaving women who believed they had been harmed by the devices few places to turn for compensation for their losses.[75]

In an effort to bring closure to the breast implant controversy, on August 25, 1997, Dow Corning offered to pay $2.4 billion to the tens of thousands of women who had filed claims against the company. Women and their attorneys immediately criticized the new proposal, claiming it was inadequate and unjust. Ed Blizzard, a lawyer for the Dow Corning bankruptcy Tort Claimants Committee, estimated that under this plan women would receive on average only $5,000—not nearly enough to cover their exorbitant medical expenses.[76] Women would have the option to refuse Dow's offer and pursue litigation on their own. However, the proposal stipulates that before such trials begin, the court must determine whether there is sufficient scientific evidence of a causal relationship between breast implants and disease. Dow has recently admitted to various complications associated with the devices, including ruptures and encapsulation; however, the company continues to argue that silicone implants do not cause debilitating autoimmune diseases.

A History of Medical Evidence [77]

The medical community has never claimed that breast implants are completely risk-free. For instance, plastic surgeons recognize that implant mammaplasty may lead to the development of infections, capsular contracture, and interfere with early tumor detection. Nevertheless, most physicians maintain the view that these complications do not pose a serious threat to women's health. Some research, however, contradicts this claim.[78] For instance, although infection is a risk common to any surgical procedure, some studies suggest that implantation procedures, in particular, pose a greater danger than other types of surgeries. Compromised surgical techniques and device sterility are factors contributing to this risk. Other studies have concluded that factors specific to breast implants may increase the risk of infection: "Staphylococcus epidermidis, which has been cultured from uninfected breast glands, may cause subclinical infections [around the breast implant] if the ductal system is disrupted during the surgical procedure."[79]

The most common implant-related risk reported in the medical literature is capsular contracture, the formation of fibrous tissue growth around the breast implant, which frequently leads to a painful hardening or distortion of the shape of the breast.[80] However, reports of contracture rates among patients have varied tremendously. For instance, the American Society of Plastic and Reconstructive Surgeons maintains in its literature that capsular contracture occurs in only 10 percent of implanted patients; whereas one implant manufacturer contends that contracture can occur in as many as 74 percent of patients receiving the device.[81] The most recent study on the complications associated with breast implants reports a 17.5 percent contracture rate.[82]

Another "known" risk associated with breast implants is the interfer-

ence with the accuracy of mammograms—a problem reported in medical journals since the 1980s. One study reported that 22–83 percent
of glandular tissue is obstructed by the presence of an implant.[83] If a
woman's breasts have hardened due to capsular contracture, a techni-
cian may not be able to compress her breast in order to take the X ray.
Given that the breast cancer rate among women in the United States is
close to 10 percent, the risk of interference with early tumor detection
could have serious consequences for a large number of patients.[84]

While the medical community has admitted that some complications
with implants do exist, they have maintained the view that there is in-
sufficient evidence linking breast implants to debilitating illnesses such
as cancer, autoimmune disease, or connective tissue disorders. In fact,
before the FDA advisory panel met in 1991 to discuss medical evidence
regarding these controversial risks, plastic surgeons launched a lobby-
ing campaign, paying for over four hundred women to fly to Washington, D.C., to tell their congressmen and senators about the importance
of breast implants to self-esteem. Plastic surgeons also contributed over
$60,000 to politicians who later wrote to the FDA commissioner advis-
ing him to keep implants on the market.[85] Despite these efforts, the
FDA restricted the distribution and use of breast implants in 1992. Position statements of the American Medical Association, the American
College of Rheumatology, the American College of Surgeons, the
American College of Radiology, the Society of Surgical Oncologists,
and the American Society of Plastic and Reconstructive Surgeons all
opposed this decision, claiming that the benefits of implants far outweigh their risks.[86] Shortly after the FDA's decision, Marcia Angell, the
executive editor of a prestigious medical journal, wrote that the decision
was unfair, claiming that women have the right to make their own
medical choices. Angell also believed that the decision caused unnecessary anxiety among women who were already implanted with the
devices.[87]

Despite the medical community's response to the FDA's 1992 decision, studies have linked breast implants or exposure to silicone to a
number of harmful, autoimmune-type side effects since the early 1960s.
These studies first appeared in Japanese medical journals after Japanese
scientists and researchers began witnessing an array of complications
and systemic problems among women who had received silicone breast
injections. Due to language and cultural barriers, findings from this
research did not reach American medical journals until the late 1970s.

In 1984, Yauo Kumagai and his colleagues published a review of the Japanese literature on the relationship between connective-tissue disease and silicone in *Arthritis and Rheumatism*.[88] The authors found that from 1964 to 1981, twenty-nine patients reported having an immune response to silicone or paraffin after they had received injections of the substances into their breasts. Thirteen of these patients were actually diagnosed with a specific connective-tissue disease. The most frequently occurring conditions among these women were scleroderma, lupus, rheumatoid arthritis, and progressive systemic sclerosis. In the same article, the authors presented their own clinical findings from a study of patients who had received silicone injections. They concluded that "prolonged exposure to [silicone] may play a role in the induction of immunological disorders."[89] This article instigated further research examining the relationship between silicone exposure and rheumatic disease. However, many of these studies were never published in medical journals.[90] Not until the late 1980s and early 1990s did research linking implants to autoimmune disease appear in the literature. These studies were published in rheumatology journals[91] as well as medical journals available to a larger audience of physicians from different specialties.[92]

Although some recent studies on implant-related risk conclude silicone can cause a systemic autoimmune response among women who have undergone breast augmentation,[93] most of the research, to date, confirms that there is not a statistically significant relationship between implants and scleroderma, rheumatoid arthritis, systemic lupus erythematosus, Sjögren's syndrome, and mixed connective tissue disease.[94] One study suggests that since patients receive biased information about connective-tissue disease and breast implants through the media, support groups, and the legal system, a conclusive study is nearly impossible.[95]

The Risk of Cancer

Another debated risk associated with breast implants is the possibility that the devices can cause cancer. The risk of cancer associated with polyurethane-foam-covered implants was discussed earlier in this chapter. Some researchers believe that silicone implants even without the polyurethane foam covering may lead to breast cancer. This conclusion stems from a number of animal studies that have shown that after rodents were injected or implanted with silicone, a significant number of them developed the disease.[96] In addition, individual case reports have suggested a link between cancer and breast augmentation with silicone.[97] Again, this evidence is contradicted by a number of studies that do not support a relationship between implants and cancer.[98] In fact, one of these studies actually concludes that women who undergo breast augmentation have less of a chance of developing breast cancer than the general population.[99]

The Risk to Exposed Children

Finally, evidence has surfaced suggesting that children of women with breast implants may be adversely affected. One study recently found that breast-feeding children of mothers with implants have a high incidence of scleroderma problems or esophageal disease.[100] If silicone particles migrate to a woman's placenta during her pregnancy, her unborn fetus may be exposed to the substance and develop similar problems after birth. One report presents two case studies of children who developed rheumatic problems after being exposed to silicone from their mothers' implants and recommends that women with breast implants refrain from breast-feeding until further data are available.[101]

Even though these studies are recent, women have been concerned for many years about the possibility that implants may cause problems in breast-feeding children. In fact, when I first began my research, I learned about a woman in Long Island, New York, who in the late 1980s had found over fifty cases of children who were afflicted with strange symptoms after they were breast-fed. All of their mothers had received implants prior to their pregnancies. Despite these cases, the American Society of Plastic and Reconstructive Surgeons states, "There is no evidence that silicones have any teratogenetic or mutagenic effect. . . . There is also no evidence that breast implants interfere with lactation, and many women with implants have successfully nursed." The position statement further reports that an anti-colic medication contains traces of silicone, implying that women should not worry if their children are exposed to the substance.[102] Even La Leche League International maintains the view that mother's milk that may be tainted with silicone is better for a child than infant formula.[103]

The history of the medical and scientific evidence regarding the risks associated with implant mammaplasty, as well as other procedures used to enhance the size of women's breasts, is an example of how medical knowledge continuously evolves and is always uncertain. Breast injections, implantable sponges, and silicone breast implants have all been associated with a number of complications and health problems. While the medical community acknowledges some of these risks (such as capsular contracture and infection), physicians have been reluctant to recognize others—especially the possibility that implants may cause women to develop debilitating autoimmune-related illnesses. Physicians and implant recipients respond to the medical uncertainty associated with breast implants in varying ways. Before addressing these issues, however, I explore the reasons women give for choosing to have the size and shape of their breasts surgically altered.

3

The Decision to Seek Breast Implants

Women's Participation in the Medicalization Process

Medicalization is a "broad definitional process" that occurs on at least three different levels: "the conceptual, the institutional and interactional levels."[1] The case of surgery involving breast implants illustrates each of these levels. First, on the conceptual level of medicalization, medical vocabulary is used to define a condition or bodily process as pathological. In the previous chapter, I described how plastic surgeons in the 1950s justified enhancing women's breasts by perceiving "small breasts" as a psychological problem for which a medical cure could be developed and employed. In turn, "micromastia" became the diagnostic label for the "disfiguring" and "pathological" condition that left women feeling inadequate, desexed, or unfeminine. Second, the institutional level of medicalization involves an organization's adopting a medical approach to treat "a particular problem in which the organization specializes."[2] The widespread use of breast implants among plastic surgeons to "cure" "diseased" or "abnormal" breasts in order to improve women's self-esteem and self-image clearly reflects this process.

The case of breast implants not only illustrates both the conceptual and institutional levels of medicalization, but also provides an example of how these two levels interact: Medical vocabulary is used not only to define "diseased" breasts, but also to describe procedures involving their treatment. Implant mammaplasty is one of the few surgeries performed on women for two seemingly different reasons—some women undergo "reconstructive" surgery with implants in order to restore their appearance following a mastectomy, while others undergo elective, or "cosmetic" implant mammaplasty in order to enhance or improve their appearance. In this chapter, I compare the experiences of women who had implants following mastectomies with those who had implants for breast enhancement in order to show how the extent to which receiving implants is perceived as a "choice" varies, depending upon how women's bodies are medically defined.

In this chapter, I also explore medicalization at the level of doctor-patient interaction, when diagnosis and treatment of a problem occurs.[3] In other words, drawing from women's descriptions of their encounters with plastic surgeons, I examine the process whereby plastic surgeons and women alike redefine healthy breasts as "pathological" based on their own preconceived notions about how a female body ought to appear.[4] While female breast size and shape have come under the medical gaze, in the end, it is *women* who decide that their breasts are in need of "treatment" with implants. In some circles, the recognition of this dimension of medicalization leads to a "blame the victim" or "they asked for it, they got it" mentality; since women willfully agree to have breast implants, if they experience side effects associated with them, it is *their* problem. This mode of thought, however, ignores the larger cultural contexts of the decision to seek implants, failing to recognize that women's own needs and motives stem from the gendered power structure of our society.

Feminist Debates on Women's Involvement with Cosmetic Surgery

Kathy Davis recognizes that with regard to cosmetic surgery, women are not merely passive victims of medicalization.[5] She writes: "Cosmetic surgery is not imposed upon women, who, blinded by the promise of a new body, meekly place their bodies under the surgeon's knife. Nor is it strictly a matter of individual choice, independent of the cultural and social practices of the beauty system. The decision to undergo cosmetic surgery is a problematic one, requiring ongoing deliberation and justification."[6] Drawing from interviews with women who either were considering, or had already undergone, cosmetic surgery, Davis explores the process through which women go about making the decision to surgically alter their bodies. A primary theme in her research addresses the role of agency—or, "the capacity of the individual to act upon her circumstances"[7]—in women's decisions to reshape their bodies. She contends that most theoretical frameworks for understanding women's beauty practices tend to focus on how such practices work to discipline and control women. For instance, the traditional feminist perspective focuses on beauty as oppression;[8] that is, women partake in beauty practices because they have internalized institutionalized patterns of gender inequality in the larger society that lull them into believing that if they change their appearance, their lives will somehow be better. More recent scholarship focuses on beauty as cultural discourse.[9] According to this framework, cultural representations of the female body are a site for exploring the interplay between gender and power relations in our larger social world. In this way the body can be read as a text that tells a story about patterns of control and ideas about femininity within broader social and historical contexts. Whether the emphasis is on beauty as oppression or as cultural discourse, these frameworks perpetuate the view of women as victims who are "blinded by consumer capitalism, oppressed by patriarchal ideologies, or inscribed within the discourses of femininity."[10] According to Davis, these models are overly simplified since they ignore how women themselves actively participate in their own decision to undergo cosmetic surgery.

Davis views women not as cultural dopes, who have been blinded by the promise of a new body; rather she perceives them as moral actors who negotiate what should and should not be done to their outward appearances. The women she spoke with were acutely aware of how media norms shaped their understanding of femininity and female attractiveness. Despite this recognition, they opted to undergo surgery to reshape their bodies anyway, believing this would alleviate their own personal suffering. Thus, Davis asserts that within a cultural context where a woman's sense of self is intrinsically linked to her bodily appearance, going under the knife is just as much a "liberating" experience as it is an oppressive one.

Like Davis, the philosopher Susan Bordo views the "old" feminist oppressive model, which theorizes men as possessing and wielding power over powerless women as inadequate for explaining women's involvement in beauty practices.[11] Drawing on Michel Foucault's conceptualization of power as a dynamic web of noncentralized forces,[12] Bordo argues that the perception of beauty as "oppressive" is "insufficiently attentive to the multiplicity of meaning, the pleasure of shaping and decorating the body, or the role of female agency in reproducing patriarchal culture."[13] Bordo also agrees with Davis that, as an *individual choice*, a woman's decision to surgically reshape her body can be perceived as liberating. It is liberating for a woman who, within certain cultural constraints, wants to make her life as gratifying and enjoyable as possible. However, criticizing Davis's approach, Bordo does not perceive cosmetic surgery as "being first and foremost 'about' self-determination or self-deception."[14] Rather, her focus is on "the complexly and densely institutionalized *system* of values and practices within which girls and women—and increasingly men and boys as well—come to believe that they are nothing (and are frequently treated as nothing) unless they are trim, tight, lineless, bulgeless, and sagless."[15]

Bordo argues that Davis's approach celebrates women's creative agency while denying the systemic patterns that shape their decisions. She supports this criticism with reflections about her own decision to lose weight through a national weight loss program in the early 1990s. In particular, Bordo discusses the message her dieting might have conveyed to the female students she teaches: Before losing weight she was able to demonstrate to these students that it is possible to be successful, confident, and expressive in a "less than normalized body"; yet, after "playing by the cultural roles" and transforming her bodily appearance, she could no longer serve as this alternative role model.[16] She explains, "Even though my choice to diet was a conscious and 'rational' response to the system of cultural meanings that surround me (not the blind submission of a 'cultural dope'), I should not deceive myself into thinking that my own feeling of enhanced personal comfort and power means that I am not servicing an oppressive system."[17] Bordo's reflection demonstrates the extent to which practices to achieve "normal" bodies can be experienced as both liberating and empowering, but still be shaped by cultural forces that perpetuate women's subordinate and objectified role in society. Her comment also suggests that women who partake in beauty regimens are not "blindly" succumbing to a cultural standard of femininity. Women know the routes to success in this culture, and are not "dopes" to pursue them. As one woman I interviewed, Sophie, explained:

The commercials, the models, the advertisements on TV—they always show beautiful women with perfect bodies with nice breasts, beautiful faces and everything. And, because of that, women believe they should look that way in order to be successful. It is true that the more attractive you are, the closer you are to success—getting the job that you like, and getting the attention of the people that you want to get attention from. Women who are more attractive and who look the stereotypical look, the ideal look, have more opportunities to get ahead.

In other words, women are fully aware of the media norms that constrain and limit their ways of thinking about female attractiveness. They also recognize that in order to "get ahead" in life, or be "successful," they must adhere to a narrowly defined cultural standard.

According to Bordo, women's participation in beauty practices reflects the intersection of complex cultural, social, and historical forces. Her research shows how consumerism and a prevailing backlash against women have perpetuated the commodification and objectification of the female body. Media images, in particular, promote an idealization of the female body, leading women who fail to adhere to homogenous representations of femininity to feel overly anxious and inadequate. I similarly argue that although women may actively and knowledgeably participate in the medicalization of femininity by choosing to alter their bodies with breast implants, their decisions are, nevertheless, rooted in a complex web of contexts that shape and perpetuate the objectification of their own bodies. Like Bordo and Davis, I do not relegate women who choose to reshape their bodies to the realm of "cultural dopes." The women I interviewed were aware of structured inequalities within the larger society as well as prevailing media norms that limited their own views of female attractiveness. They did not simply opt for a beauty change because they had been taken in by ideal images of femininity on television commercials, or in magazine advertisements that displayed thin, perfectly proportioned female bodies. However, most of the women I spoke with did not perceive their decision to seek implants as a "liberating" or "empowering" experience. Rather, nearly half of the women I interviewed, in hindsight, came to view their "choice" to undergo surgery as one made under specific pressure from significant others in their lives who had convinced them that they would be more worthy of love and attention if they adhered to cultural norms of femininity.

Opting for Breast Enhancement:
The Influence of Interpersonal Relationships

Researchers and scholars have noted the significance of relationships in women's decisions to undergo cosmetic surgery. For instance, Susan Bordo suggests that women who seek breast implants are not passively taken in by the cultural image of the "beautiful breast," but have correctly discerned that this image "shapes the perceptions and desires of potential lovers and employers."[18] Similarly, Diana Dull and Candace West examined the reasons why women undergo cosmetic surgery and found that family members, peers, and employers influence women's desire for aesthetic improvement.[19] Contrary to these findings, Davis discovered in her research that women felt pressure from family, spouses, and friends *not* to undergo cosmetic surgery. These significant others in women's lives tried to persuade them that they did not need to adhere to a false cultural ideal in order to be valued. Nevertheless, Davis's respondents opted for surgery anyway. Consequently, their descriptions of their reasons for reshaping their bodies were triumphant accounts of overcoming resistance. They viewed their decision to have surgery as "empowering"—they were finally taking the action necessary to alleviate their personal suffering.[20]

A few of the women I interviewed who decided to have breast implants also perceived this decision as, in a sense, liberating. For instance, Sarah, who had her breast implants when she was twenty years old because her breasts appeared "tubular," explained that she felt extremely uncomfortable and self-conscious about her body. Receiving implants was a decision she made, under her own free will, to eliminate her personal feelings of inadequacy: "I, at the time, had no boyfriend. . . . I mean the choice was something that—that is what I wanted to do when I was young. I knew I didn't look right. Something wasn't normal in comparison to other girls that I had seen. So, that was the reason for me. No one else influenced me at all." Similarly, Carmen decided to receive breast implants because she "admired breasts" and was simply tired of having ones that were "so tiny." Even though Carmen's mother tried to persuade her not to go through with cosmetic surgery, Carmen made an appointment with a plastic surgeon anyway. She explained, "I was the only one who made [my small breast size] an issue. Being a woman, I just like breasts and felt like I got ripped off. . . . It came to a point when I just got fed up. You know, I know that some women do it for other men, maybe to get attention, but I got attention without my implants. I did it for myself."

Despite these remarks, most of the women I spoke with who opted to undergo surgery to enhance the size and shape of their breasts explained that they did not choose implants "for themselves." Contrary to Davis's findings, these women did not perceive their decision as an "empowering" experience or as a way to take hold of their lives. Rather, nearly 70 percent of the women in my study who had implants for "cosmetic" purposes perceived this decision as an action taken under specific interpersonal pressure. The nature of women's relationships with lovers, spouses, peers, and family members strongly influenced the ways in which they thought about their own bodies, leading them to plastic surgeons' offices. While these women were not culturally "duped," they were not enthusiastically opting for surgical breast enhancement; their descriptions of their interpersonal relationships suggest that they were reluctantly succumbing to ideal beauty standards to please significant others in their lives. For instance, Christine explained that no one had forced her into having her breasts enlarged, but the nature of her relationship with her husband was such that she felt pressure to go through with the surgery. Twenty-six years previously, when Christine was twenty-nine, she actually thought that breast enhancement would save her marriage:

> My husband and I were going through a divorce and I asked him what the problem was, because our sex life wasn't very good and we were having problems. And he said, "Well, you don't have the figure that you had when I married you." And I said, "Well, what do you mean?" He said, "Well, your breasts are so saggy." (This is after two children.) So, I had decided to divorce him and then I had second thoughts. I thought maybe I should give my best effort. . . . I think I felt that if my husband didn't want me this way, no other man would want me.

Christine did not receive implants solely "for herself." She viewed her decision to reshape her body as an effort made to please her husband, who no longer found her attractive.

Leslie, who received breast implants fifteen years ago when she was nineteen years old, also linked her negative self-image to her relationship with her husband:

> I didn't know at the time how heavily [my ex-husband] had influenced my brain. I probably, in retrospect, had a very poor self-image. Because of being

the type of controlling person that he was, he was probably able to play those things against myself to—I don't know—maybe make me believe that [receiving implants] would be something that would be good for me. He used to make fun of parts of my body. . . . And, he made me believe that if I was ever to go anywhere or leave him, no one would have anything to do with me because I was this deformed type of person. That is the only reason I could think of as to why I possibly [got the implants].

Believing that her husband's comments about her body were valid and that nobody would desire her the way she appeared, Leslie chose cosmetic surgery. Both Christine and Leslie's descriptions of their relationships with their spouses indicate that they did not perceive their decision to reshape their bodies as an act of self-determination, or as a means to exercise their freedom of choice about how they, themselves, wanted to present themselves to the world. Hoping to improve their marriages, they were simply succumbing to their husbands' wishes.

Sheila described two factors that contributed to her decision to have her breasts surgically enhanced: first, a distorted sense of self and body image and, second, her spouse's constant ridicule of her appearance. Sheila had received breast implants in 1973, when she was twenty-nine. At the time, she was married, had two children, and was actively pursuing a career in retail. In the 1970s, many young women, like Sheila, were exploring meaningful careers outside the home; however, they also were continuing to maintain their role as primary caretaker within the family. Trying to "have it all," Sheila explained, took its toll on her self-esteem:

Back then, I was having a hard time dealing with me for who I really was. . . . I wasn't happy with myself. . . . It was during the time when Gloria Steinem was running around. I didn't want to be staying at home watching Phil Donahue, you know, and taking care of the kids all day long. . . . And then, you know, many women were running around just wanting to have it all. So, that was a very frustrating time—women in general were a mess, a total mess.

Already confused about her own sense of identity during a time when the meaning of womanhood was under radical reconstruction, Sheila's husband contributed to her troubles. In particular, his constant ridicule of her bodily appearance made her feel inadequate and unfeminine, leading her to visit a plastic surgeon:

I felt very self-conscious. I didn't feel as good about myself as I guess I should have. Basically, [receiving implants] was to fulfill an emotional need to feel better about myself. Therapy was out of the question. I was twenty-eight or twenty-nine—so, you don't think in terms—you think well, you just get it fixed. You don't think there is a deeper problem. And my ex-husband used to tease me a lot. Which, I am not blaming him, but I would say there lies a problem. I mean, it bothered me. I felt self-conscious and instead of turning around and just saying, "Well, your toes are stupid" or something, you know, I let it affect me and I decided to do something about it.

Rather than seek counseling to understand the source of her poor self-esteem, Sheila relied on medicine to provide her with a quick and simple "fix" for her suffering. Indeed, she perceived her decision to undergo cosmetic surgery, at the time, as the best course of action to alleviate her own personal and emotional pain. However, her descriptions of the social and cultural contexts that shaped her reason for undergoing cosmetic surgery suggest that she eventually came to believe that her decision to have her breasts enlarged was rooted in her confusion about her "expected" role as a woman, as well as her relationship with her husband, who teased her about the way she appeared.

The descriptions of the social contexts that led Sheila, Leslie, Christine, and other women I interviewed to receive breast implants indicate that not all women perceive themselves as active agents who feel empowered by their decision to surgically alter their appearances. These women did not have breast implants "for themselves"; rather, their decision to enhance the size of their breasts was made under specific pressure from husbands who had internalized a cultural link between ideal femininity and breast size. Lorraine, for instance, had implants because her husband seemed to think that she was "too small and jiggled" after having her son. She believed that his obsession with breasts was linked to larger cultural forces: "I think it all started with that damn *Playboy* magazine. The epitome of the girl next-door. You know, the big breasts . . . and this is every man's dream, and this is how she is supposed to look and, if she doesn't, then 'Hey guys, we have stuff to fix her up!' And, I feel very strongly that that type of thinking was imparted to my husband."

If female breasts are a cultural indicator of femininity, it makes sense that in order for some men to feel more "masculine," they would want their female counterparts to have bigger, more shapely breasts. As Susan Brownmiller writes: "Femininity pleases men because it makes them appear more masculine by contrast; and, in truth, conferring an extra portion of unearned gender distinction on men, an unchallenged space in which to breathe freely and feel stronger, wiser, more competent, is femininity's special gift."[21] Not surprisingly, most of the women I interviewed who felt pressured into receiving implants reported that a male lover or husband were the ones who had convinced them that they would be "better off" if they had larger breasts. A few, however, explained that their own parents had influenced their decision to undergo cosmetic surgery. Joyce, for example, elaborated on how her upbringing had influenced her own sense of self and body image.

Upon first impression, Joyce appeared to have a comfortable and stable life. She is a thirty-year-old, middle-class white woman, who is married and has two children, ages four and nine. The house in which she and her family live is in a suburban neighborhood where I could envision summer block parties and children playing hockey or soccer in the streets as common occurrences. Joyce is currently a homemaker and her husband has been employed by the government for over ten years—a job that is both "steady and secure."

Despite the cheerful exterior, throughout the course of my three-hour interview with Joyce, I gradually learned that her life had not always been so comfortable and settled. Joyce grew up in what she referred to as an extremely "dysfunctional" household. Both of her parents suffered from mental illness; her father was diagnosed with schizophrenia, and her mother had a long history of depression. As a consequence, Joyce explained, neither parent was able to provide her with the encouragement, support, and attention that she needed while growing up. Emotionally tormented by her father, who constantly reinforced the notion that "men are the kings and women are worthless and useless," and ignored by her docile and passive mother, Joyce decided to run away from home when she was nine years old. Feeling inadequate and deficient, she spent her adolescent years moving back and forth from the streets to juvenile detention facilities.

Despite her troubled past, by the time Joyce turned twenty, her life had improved immensely. She had found a decent-paying job as a hairdresser and had fallen in love with the man she later married. Nevertheless, Joyce explained that the emotional scars from her past had never healed—she continued to feel somehow "less than" and "different" from other women her age. Her belief that her body appeared less than ideal contributed to her low self-esteem and lack of self-confidence. In particular, Joyce explained that her breasts sagged after nursing her son, and that she had a benign tumor removed from her right breast which left her "kind of lopsided." Joyce was so embarrassed and ashamed about her bodily appearance that she would cross out bra advertisements with a black marker in the Sunday paper, because seeing bodies that appeared "so perfect" made her "emotionally sick." To alleviate her suffering, in 1982, at the age of twenty-five, Joyce decided to undergo cosmetic surgery, to uplift her breasts and make them larger and more symmetrical.

Believing that one's "view of femininity comes from what one is told while growing up," Joyce felt that her decision to seek breast implants stemmed from a combination of two forces: "a society that puts pictures of perfect women in your face constantly," and her relationship with her parents—specifically her father, who perpetuated her belief that a woman's only attribute is her bodily appearance. For Joyce, "having implants was a way to make all the pain go away." She perceived her decision to undergo this surgery as the best course of action to alleviate her own personal suffering. However, her description of the source of her pain suggests that this action was largely influenced by the oppressive nature of her familial relationships and the gendered culture in which women's bodies are exploited and objectified.

Like Joyce, Ann also believed that her decision to receive breast implants twenty years ago was influenced by her relationship with her father, who would "always give these throwaway comments like 'Oh there is this lady, she is very nice—flat as a pancake—but so nice.'" After spending her childhood in an environment where her value as a woman was linked to her breast size, in her late teens, Ann moved to southern California, "a world full of body beautifuls." This new environment further reinforced her belief that "if you are attractive, you are loved—if you are not, you are invalidated." Following her move, a female acquaintance explained to her, "You really are pretty attractive, except if you just had bigger boobs." Soon thereafter, Ann began to entertain the idea of undergoing cosmetic surgery to enlarge her breasts. Her father's reaction to this thought "sealed the deal" for her: "We were driving, just [me and my father] and he stopped the car. And, he said to me, 'Your mother told me you were thinking about [getting implants] and I want to tell you that I think it is a great idea. I wish she would do it. Whatever man you are with, he is really going to like that a lot.'" Because, at the time, Ann's "sense of self just wasn't there," she was unable to separate her father's misconstrued perceptions about female bodily appearances from her own ideas about what makes a woman "feminine." As a result, her father's reaction to her wish to receive implants reinforced her belief that if she had larger breasts, she would be more worthy of a fulfilling, happier life.

Similarly, Alice explained that when she received implants, she was "behaving in a very unconscious mode." Only in hindsight did she realize that her reason for seeking cosmetic surgery was related to her hidden desire to relive her adolescence: "Having plastic surgery meant for me that I could go back and be that pretty teenager that I never felt I was and get the love, and get the boyfriends—and just get through that period of life. Because, when I was a teenager, I was chubby. Furthermore, I didn't like being so Italian-looking because I was in a high school full of these tall blondes in the late sixties, early seventies—you had to be skinny like Twiggy." Alice explained that her father had reinforced her feelings of inadequacy when she was growing up: "My father was one of those rage-aholics who was not very warm and loving and affectionate. He was a highly critical person . . . never quite approving of me—of anything in regards to—he was just highly dysfunctional, unhappy, miserable, depressed—an angry human being. . . . I grew up feeling extremely inadequate—not terribly bright. I never had any confidence with my intelligence, nor with my bodily appearance."

Not only do fathers fulfill their roles as socializers, teaching their daughters that they would be better off in life if they adhered to traditional standards of femininity and female attractiveness, but mothers, too, "sense that good looks may be the most important legacy they can pass on to a young girl. It is the mother's magic wand, an insurance policy to guarantee happiness ever after."[22] While some of the women I interviewed claimed that their relationships with their fathers influenced their decision to seek breast implants, others believed that their interactions with their mothers shaped this decision. Hillary recalled: "I guess for me, my mother was very attractive and she kind of—because, I was overweight—she taught me to believe that when I got thin and looked good, then everything was going to be perfect. For me, I think it was probably a perfection issue which kind of played into me getting [the implants] in the first place."

In Karen's case, her mother gave her breast implants as an eighteenth-birthday present. Karen had felt very self-conscious about feeling small-breasted, and her mother (who also had received implants) thought that having larger breasts would boost her self-esteem. Describing her family, Karen provided insights into how her mother may have influenced her decision to receive implants: "I came from a very externally oriented family, [that placed] too much focus on the outside, too much focus on appearances, usually what we consider 'perfect.' My family was very conscious about body image, as I was. . . . At the time I thought [getting implants] was a great idea. I was in favor of it. In hindsight, I think I did it more because my mother thought it was a good idea." Years after she had her surgery, Karen realized that her mother conflated her low self-esteem with her bodily appearance, which did not "fit" with the ideal standard of female attractiveness.

Beth also believed that her mother influenced her desire for larger breasts: "My mother would tease me and, when I was a teenager, call my breasts mosquito bites. You know, maybe it was endearing on her part but, for me, I didn't—I wasn't aware enough to really ask her why she had called [them] that. I just sort of made it up in my own mind that I was inferior. So, I think that is really where my low self-esteem started." Ideas about female attractiveness, sexuality, and breast size and shape are socially constructed through a process whereby social institutions like the media perpetuate images of the "attractive" woman as thin with perfectly proportioned bodies. These depictions, in turn, shape the basis for what is valued in our society to the extent that when a woman's breast size or shape falls short of the cultural representation of femininity, she feels that something in her life is drastically missing. Mona explained, "There is a subtle message, this facade that we are supposed to be applying ourselves to. And, it feels lacking. So, we all do some searching to fulfill something that might make us feel more whole." For many of the women I interviewed, receiving breast implants was a means to fill this void in their lives; many believed that having larger breasts would improve their relationships with spouses and lovers; others were convinced by their own parents and peers that reshaping their bodies would inevitably enable them to lead richer, fuller lives. In hindsight, these women recognized that at the root of their desire to have larger or more shapely breasts were deeper problems associated with the nature of their interpersonal relationships.

The personal and social contexts that shaped my respondents' decision to seek breast implants indicate that women's participation in medicalization is less a reflection of their capacity to take hold of their lives and exercise their freedom of choice than it is a manifestation of the specific nature of their own subordination. Many of the women I interviewed had years to reflect on their lives before and after receiving breast implants. This time enabled them to understand how their interpersonal relationships served as threads linking the macro, gendered structure of American society to their own micro, day-to-day feelings about themselves and about their bodies. Women's spouses, peers, parents, and lovers had internalized the societal message that women are more worthy of love and attention when they adhere to a narrowly defined cultural image of femininity. Through critical comments or passing remarks, these friends, lovers, spouses, and family members conveyed this message to the women I interviewed, who, themselves, began to believe that their lives would improve if they changed their appearances. Thus, they reluctantly chose to undergo cosmetic surgery.

Becoming a "Good Candidate" for Breast Augmentation

Despite the wide range of outside influences affecting the decision to receive breast implants, plastic surgeons claim that cosmetic surgery is appropriate only for women who think surgery will improve their self-esteem and improve their self-image. It is not recommended for women who think it will help them "attract a younger lover or maintain their spouse's attention."[23] These definitions of "good" and "bad" candidates for cosmetic surgery ignore the connection many women experience between their own feelings of self-worth and their relationships with certain men. Moreover, the two definitions obscure the complex and oppressive nature of the cultural and interpersonal contexts that shape women's ideas about their bodily appearance.[24] Even when my respondents claimed that they were undergoing surgery "for themselves," throughout the course of my interviews with them, they gradually revealed outside influences that had played a part in their opting for cosmetic surgical alteration. For instance, Georgine explained that no one in particular had influenced her decision to seek breast implants. She simply knew that in her line of business (modeling), having small breasts hindered her career. She also assumed that having larger breasts would be "more pleasing for [her] husband to look at" and that implants would provide her with "something better to offer him." Implicit in her descriptions of the factors shaping her decision to receive implants is the cultural belief that in order for a woman to be valued, she must adhere to an ideal of femininity that is characterized by a body with large breasts. Perceiving her implants as a kind of "gift" for her husband, Georgine suggests that one way for a woman to receive more love and attention from a man is to enhance her breast size. Plastic surgeons hold the power to perpetuate the idea that a woman's self-worth is connected to her outward bodily appearance by providing her with a quick surgical solution for feelings of inadequacy and undesirability.

According to Diana Dull and Candace West, cosmetic surgery is inherently problematic since plastic surgeons are always entering into a realm clearly beyond the medical mandate to define the nature and treatment of disease.[25] In other words, plastic surgeons continually construct appearances and perform surgery that, by its own definition, is unnecessary. In an effort to understand how plastic surgeons legitimize the procedures they perform, and how people who elect such surgeries make sense of their decisions to do so, Dull and West conducted interviews with plastic surgeons and their prospective patients. They discovered that the construction of "good candidates" for cosmetic surgery not only involves plastic surgeons choosing patients who seek cosmetic surgery "for themselves," but also involves the "accomplishment of gender." That is, surgeons and patients perceive cosmetic surgery as "normal" and "natural" for women, but not for men. In effect, when women visit their plastic surgeons, *cosmetic* surgery inevitably becomes a *reconstructive* undertaking through a process whereby patients and surgeons alike redefine normal, female bodily features as "'flaws,' 'defects,' 'deformities,' and 'correctable problems' of appearance."[26] This process of redefinition enables surgeons to justify their activities while allowing those who elect cosmetic surgery to make rational sense of their decision to do so.

Women turn to plastic surgeons because they are unhappy with the size or shape of a part of their body. In turn, plastic surgeons have a preconceived notion of how a woman's body *ought* to appear and are able to shape definitions of desirable gendered traits. My findings concur with those presented in the research of Dull and West. Over a quarter of the women I spoke with who had breast implants for "cosmetic" reasons explained that their plastic surgeons' opinions about how their bodies *ought* to appear influenced their decision to receive breast implants. Women's plastic surgeons justified their surgeries through a process of labeling their normal, healthy breasts as "defective" and "flawed." In turn, women became "good candidates" for implant mammaplasty.

Mona explained that before undergoing cosmetic surgery her breasts were slightly asymmetrical. Unaware that "not all women have breasts which are the same size," she felt abnormal and unfeminine. Her husband, who used to "make comments about women and their figures," made her feel especially uncomfortable and embarrassed about the way her body appeared. To alleviate her suffering, Mona decided to visit a plastic surgeon, who told her that "because [she] had one breast that was smaller than the other," she was an "ideal candidate" for receiving breast implants. Although Mona felt that her surgeon did not encourage or influence her decision to seek breast implants, her case illustrates how plastic surgeons legitimize cosmetic surgery involving implants by labeling some women as more *in need* of surgery than others. This label is dependent upon plastic surgeons' own preconceptions of female bodily appearance. Even though, years after her cosmetic surgery, Mona realized that having two breasts of different sizes is a common phenomenon, in American culture this asymmetry is not perceived as "normal." Plastic surgeons convey this type of message to their patients, deciding that bodily alterations are more necessary for some women than for others.

Implantation as a "Quick and Easy Solution"

One surgeon explained to a woman I interviewed, "I like doing breast implants. They are the biggest part of my practice because it is really easy: Cut it open, put it in—it's like changing a tire." Other cosmetic procedures performed on the breast are not as simple, but require a great deal more time and skill. For instance, the "flap" procedure to enlarge women's breasts entails skillfully shifting tissue from a woman's abdominal area into her chest region. Breast reduction is also complicated—if not done carefully, a woman may be left severely scarred since the surgery involves making many precise, delicate incisions in order to remove excess, fatty breast tissue.

Surprisingly, many of the women I interviewed explained that they had visited their plastic surgeons without the intention of having their breasts enlarged. Some women, for instance, were left with sagging breasts after nursing and simply wanted a "lift," which requires a procedure similar to that used to reduce the size of women's breasts—a mastopexy. Other women who had asymmetrical breasts were more concerned about their lopsided appearance than about their breast size. Nevertheless, several of the women I interviewed explained that when they visited their plastic surgeons, they became convinced that breast lifts or reductions were time-consuming and difficult procedures. During these visits, surgeons also conveyed to women the message that they would be "better off" if they conformed to a cultural ideal of female attractiveness, which is characterized by large breasts. Given all alternatives, breast augmentation was presented to many of these women as the quickest, simplest solution to their perceived problems. Christine, for example, recalled: "I went to a plastic surgeon, and he said, well, he couldn't lift my breasts—all he could do was put these implants in. I just wanted him to lift it and he told me that wasn't possible. (I later learned that it was possible.) But, he said that this was the easiest way to do it." Jane also went to see a plastic surgeon because after nursing her two children she had large, "pendulous" breasts. She, in fact, asked her physician if he could perform a breast reduction on her. She described her interaction with her surgeon as follows:

> When I went in, the doctor said, "Well, [breast reduction] is really serious surgery.... What about breast implants?"
> I said, "Well, then I would just have big boobs that hang down to my waist."
> He said, "No, no what [the implants] would do is fill in the space—they would pull your breasts up to where they are supposed to be.... Basically the problem is you don't have anything in there. You just have extra skin.... If you have the [reduction] there are more scars—it is major surgery, you know, it is more difficult to recover.... If you have the implant put in, we would make a small slit, we stuff the implant in there—you go home the same day. It's no big deal."

Convinced that her breasts were not where they were "supposed to be" and that surgery involving implants was less complicated and produced a better cosmetic result than breast reduction, Jane opted to receive a set of breast implants.

A similar case is Alice, whose breasts "sort of flattened out and drooped" in her mid-thirties. She went to visit a plastic surgeon inquiring about a "lift": "I told the doctor, 'You know, I'd like to have [my breasts] lifted.' And he goes, 'Oh, no, no, no. I could do even better for you. I could lift them without any scars because if I lifted them, you would have scars and that is really ugly and you don't want to have scars that won't go away.' (That was a lie. I didn't know it was a lie [then].)" Alice later discovered that, in fact, some plastic surgeons specialize in performing mastopexies and are trained to leave only faint, unnoticeable scars on their patients. Nevertheless, her own plastic surgeon convinced her that aside from surgery with breast implants, other cosmetic breast procedures are complicated and frequently leave "undesirable results." According to him, the benefits of having a flawless, scarless chest and a "beautiful body" with the surgical insertion of two breast implants far outweighed the disadvantages he linked with other surgical procedures.

Getting Caught Up in "Plastic Surgery Promises"

Jenna explained that she had no intention of receiving breast implants until her initial encounter with a plastic surgeon. Feeling a lot of shame about the pendulous shape of her breasts after she had nursed her three children, she visited a plastic surgeon to see if he could somehow "lift" her sagging breast tissue. However, her plastic surgeon responded to this inquiry saying, "No, no you don't want a lift, you will be too flat— you won't like it." Even though Jenna did not visit this physician to discuss increasing the size of her breasts, she began entertaining the idea of implantation: "You are so vulnerable. I mean, you are going to someone about your breasts—right? That is so—you are so vulnerable, you are just like wide open. And they tell you, 'That won't look good, that won't look good,' and you are thinking, 'Well, that is a man talking.' It is this whole spell you get under of plastic surgery promises." Jenna's comment illustrates how cultural assumptions about women as inferior and subordinate to men in the larger society transcend medical encounters.[27] The prevailing idea that a woman's primary role is to please and satisfy men has led many American women to judge themselves based on how men respond to their physical appearance. Jenna's plastic surgeon was able to lull her into believing that she would be better off (or more worthy of love and attention) because he was a "man." During this initial encounter with this surgeon, Jenna explained that he proceeded to take her breasts and squeeze them together while telling her, "Look how good [the implants] will look in a bathing suit." At that point, Jenna realized that cosmetic surgery was "more an issue about what [her plastic surgeon] thought was attractive and sexual than what [she] thought." Nevertheless, she went through with the surgery anyway.

Jenna's experience with her plastic surgeon illustrates how women's ideas about how their bodies should look may diverge from plastic surgeons' conceptions of the ideal female body. Nevertheless, plastic surgeons are perceived both as "medical experts" who know what is best for their patients and as "artists" who possess the skills necessary to construct ideal gendered traits, and they hold the power to influence a woman's decision to undergo cosmetic surgery.

From Cosmetic to Reconstructive Undertakings: Becoming "Medically Necessary"

Eleanor also had no intention of receiving breast implants when she visited her plastic surgeon. She explained that she had lost a tremendous amount of weight, leaving her with excess skin around her abdomen, and she thought a surgeon might be able to give her a simple "tuck." However, after meeting with a plastic surgeon, she was convinced that she needed not only abdominal surgery, but also breast reconstruction. Eleanor described her initial interaction with her plastic surgeon as follows: "Upon examining [my abdomen] the surgeon said to me when he looked at my breasts, 'You don't have to look like that.' My breasts were abnormal, deformed looking—they just were totally not normal looking. So, that is how it all started. When he said that you don't have to look like that, I bought it. And [this surgeon] was drop-dead gorgeous." Eleanor's plastic surgeon suggested that while he was "fixing" her abdomen, he could also provide her with breast implants, free of charge: "[Receiving implants] wasn't going to cost me anymore because—I got two [surgeries, the abdominal and breast] for the price of one. I felt like he was saying, 'Hey, I tell you what I am going to do—I got a deal for you—two for one!'" In Eleanor's case, a cosmetic procedure literally became a reconstructive undertaking—the surgeon labeled the procedure as "medically necessary" and was subsequently reimbursed by Eleanor's insurance company.

Both Jenna and Eleanor explained that their surgeons were "attractive" men who could make them "look beautiful." The combination of these factors influenced both patients' decisions to undergo surgery, demonstrating not only how gendered assumptions infiltrate plastic surgeons' ideas about what constitutes a beautiful female body, but also how women's own self-worth is deeply connected to men's responses to their physical appearances. While plastic surgeons may have the ability to construct ideal gendered traits, women become caught up in their surgical promises because they trust medical experts and assume them to be knowledgeable about what constitutes bodily perfection. The primary difference between Jenna's and Eleanor's accounts is that Jenna's surgery was deemed "cosmetic" and was not reimbursed by her insurance company, while Eleanor's surgery was considered "reconstructive" and "medically necessary." These labels allowed for third-party reimbursement. In general, "attributing a procedure to physical malfunction tends to confer the 'necessary' label on surgery, whereas socioemotional motivations are demeaned."[28] However, the case of implant mammaplasty illustrates an interesting contradiction between "necessary" and "unnecessary" surgical procedures, since implantation is nearly always provided to women who are suffering emotionally and rarely to women who need the procedure to improve physical function.

Grace's case further illuminates this dilemma. She had scoliosis, a spinal deformity that, when corrected, left her breasts asymmetrical. When she visited a plastic surgeon's office, she had no intention of receiving breast implants but was wondering if her larger breast could be reduced to match the size of her smaller one. However, when her plastic surgeon looked at the disparity between her two breasts he replied, "We will just put an implant in [the smaller one]." Grace explained that when her surgeon saw her "deformity," "he became more the artist— he wanted to create." His eagerness and desire to mold and reshape her body convinced her that she should have an implant inserted into her smaller breast. Because her surgeon perceived the asymmetry of her breasts as a "deformity," he fought with her insurance company to cover the cost of implantation. As Grace explained, "According to him, [the surgery] wasn't 'cosmetic'—he felt that it had impeded me socially." Her surgeon felt so strongly that Grace's surgery was necessary that he persuaded her insurance company to provide reimbursement. In fact, Grace became the first woman in the state where she lives to receive full compensation for breast "reconstruction" following a spinal deformity.

The labels "reconstructive" and "cosmetic" imply a clear-cut distinction between surgery that is "necessary" and surgery that is "unnecessary." The American Society of Plastic and Reconstructive Surgeons defines cosmetic surgery as a procedure "performed to reshape normal structures of the body in order to improve the patient's appearance and self-esteem."[29] While cosmetic surgery is considered "elective," in most cases, surgery deemed to be "reconstructive" is thought of as "necessary," since it is intended to restore an individual's health or physical function. Such labeling has implications for women who receive breast implants since insurance companies reimburse only for surgeries that are medically necessary or, in the case of implant mammaplasty, "reconstructive." However, whether considered cosmetic or reconstructive, in either case, receiving implants does not restore a woman's physical function or her health. Rather, the necessity of surgery is entirely dependent upon the determination of how "diseased" or "deformed" a woman's breast appears. Even though a dichotomy exists in definitional terms between procedures to alter "healthy" and "diseased" breasts, in reality, a continuum more accurately describes the situation. Women who wish to replace a breast after a mastectomy fall clearly on the "reconstructive" end of the spectrum, while women who wish implants to enlarge their small breasts fall clearly on the "cosmetic" side. The interaction between women who wish to surgically alter their "sagging" or "asymmetrical" breasts and their plastic surgeons illustrates how some surgical procedures involving breast implants do not fit neatly into "reconstructive" and "cosmetic" categories. Rather, in these cases, a gray area exists in which plastic surgeons themselves must decide on the medical necessity of breast implantation depending on their own ideas about how a woman's body ought to appear.[30] The gray-area cases described in this section show how the decision for or against surgery in general and breast implantation in particular is a social construct—surgery is classified by physicians and third-party payers as "justifiable," "urgent," or "elective," depending on economical and political considerations,[31] as well as on cultural ideals of the female body.

The Other End of the Spectrum: "Reconstructive" Surgery Following Mastectomies[32]

The feminist poet and writer Audre Lorde suggests that since the only function of breast reconstruction is to restore a woman's physical appearance, a mastectomy and the replacement of a lost breast may both be viewed as *cosmetic* occurrences.[33] Perceived as such, women who feel angry and depressed when they are faced with losing one or both of their breasts are often made to feel unacceptably vain—they are "encouraged to become detached and to 'take it like a man.'"[34] For instance, Suzanne explained that she was terribly saddened by the prospect of losing both of her breasts prior to her bilateral mastectomy; not only was she facing the imminent loss of a part of her body, but also a part of her self and her sensuality: "My breasts connect with the world like the rest of my body connects with the world. I am a very sensuous person and when I am happy, my breasts are there. So, for me, losing my breasts wasn't just about sexuality and aesthetics. For me it was truly losing a part of my body that responds and enjoys the world." Despite the meaning Suzanne attached to her breasts, she explained that one of her physicians ("an older woman in her mid- to late fifties") responded to her fears and concerns by telling her, "Dear, you know, if women were as concerned about other parts as they are about their breasts— they wouldn't have to think about these things." Suzanne interpreted this comment to mean that most women are too concerned about their bodily appearance and not concerned enough about their health in general. Suzanne found the tone of the comment patronizing and was surprised that a female physician had completely failed to understand the loss that she was about to endure.

Indeed, several of the women I interviewed who had received breast implants following a mastectomy felt that their breasts were linked to some aspect of their female identity. Rebecca explained that after her mastectomy and before her reconstructive surgery, she felt as though her missing breasts symbolized the loss of a "nurturing" side of her self that was deeply connected to her sense of womanhood: "When I lost my breasts—they are such a central part of being a woman. It was a loss. . . . My chest felt very strange and I can remember holding babies, and it was such a strange feeling because you don't have the soft mound for the baby to lay their head on." Mary, who was diagnosed with breast cancer in 1986, when she was sixty-four, also believed that losing her breasts represented a loss of femininity: "I still wanted to look my best—staying slim, dressing properly. I am from the wear-those-hats-and-white-gloves generation, you know. . . . And, so, breasts are a feminine part of us. As soon as I learned I was going to lose them, I wanted them back."

Comments such as these reflect and reinforce the idea that a woman who is diagnosed with breast cancer is confronted with the "sharp double edge of facing a potentially fatal disease, and of losing a precious part of her body that is deeply tangled in her sexuality/femininity/identity."[35] In effect, breast cancer and the subsequent loss of a breast is "assumed to produce special problems over and above those experienced by other cancer patients—specifically in the realm of sexuality and body image."[36] Responding to the cultural message that a woman's identity is intrinsically related to the presence of her breast(s), health care professionals base their recommendations for helping breast cancer patients on the presumption that every woman defines herself in terms of her bodily appearance. For example, volunteers from the American Cancer Society encourage women to try on prostheses soon after their mastectomies, conveying the message that "[women who wear prostheses] are just as good as [they] were before because [they] can look exactly the same."[37] Similarly, most medical literature recommends that women who have had their breasts surgically removed be fitted immediately with these uncomfortable devices "so that external appearance can be restored."[38] Moreover, some women are encouraged by physicians to choose a surgical solution for their perceived problem. Serving to replace their actual breasts with shiny bags filled with silicone or saline, breast reconstruction with implants has been described as the "ultimate in breast objectification."[39] The feminist theorist Iris Young suggests that such recommendations teach women that they must hide their pain and sorrow associated with their loss. Moreover, they convey the message to women that bodies without breasts are "deformed," "diseased," and "repulsive" to look at:

> Whether [a woman] wears a prosthesis or a surgically constructed artificial breast, she certainly cannot feel the same. Both objects serve to hide and deny her loss of feeling and sensitivity, both sexual and also the simple daily feeling of being in the world with these breasts. Prosthesis and reconstruction give primacy to the look, to the visual constitution of a woman's body. Her trauma is constructed not as the severance of her self and her loss of feeling, but as her becoming visually deformed, repulsive to look at. She must protect others from viewing her deformity and herself from the gaze of repulsion.[40]

Similarly, Audre Lorde claims that the decision to seek any kind of breast prosthesis after cancer is based on how women "look and feel to others, rather than how [they] feel to [themselves]."[41]

In Lorde's moving and personal account of her experience with breast cancer, she describes her own struggle to accept her body despite disfigurement. Coming to the realization that she was no less of a woman or sexual being without a breast, she chose not to wear any type of prosthesis after her mastectomy, since such devices merely offer "the empty comfort of 'nobody will know the difference.'"[42] Many of the women I interviewed who had mastectomies felt that the social scrutiny associated with the appearance of a lopsided or concave chest was all too powerful to follow the same course of action. For instance, Abby, who had reconstructive surgery after losing a breast to cancer when she was twenty-seven years old, explained, "When Dave Dravecky lost his arm to cancer, he was accepted. He walked around with one arm, people felt sorry. A woman who has lost her breast because—I can't go out on the street and walk around with one breast because I would get stared at like a freak." Other women I interviewed who had not experienced breast cancer, nevertheless, understood the social ridicule linked with the absence of a breast. Christine remarked, "If somebody has lost an arm, they would deal with it. But, you lose a breast and all of a sudden you are not a woman anymore."

In a cultural context in which a woman's breast is deeply connected with her sense of femininity and sexuality, many physicians assume that women who have just undergone a mastectomy will immediately want to restore their physical appearance. Paula reported, "My [oncologist] right away started talking about reconstruction to make me feel better. So I went to a friend of his, a plastic surgeon around the corner. So, even before I had the mastectomy, I had seen a plastic surgeon." Mary similarly stated, "Well, I received implants because I had cancer and I had to have a double mastectomy and so the surgeon sent me to a plastic surgeon. So, I just didn't consider anything else." Assuming she had no choice in the matter, Mary agreed to undergo reconstructive surgery with no questions asked.

Some evidence clearly suggests that breast reconstruction immediately following a mastectomy has a positive influence on women's self-concept. Women who are confronted with the loss of one or both of their breasts are described in the psychological literature as depressed over their impending physical loss as well as the dramatic change in their body images. The literature also suggests that these women often feel shameful, inadequate, and fearful of sexual rejection. For some, breast reconstruction helps "to alleviate such feelings and encourages women to have a more hopeful outlook."[43] Breast reconstruction following a mastectomy not only is intended to restore women's "femininity," but also her "normal" and "natural" appearance. But, sometimes, oncologists and plastic surgeons go to radical extremes to make women look "as good as new."

Kate's oncologist recommended that she visit a plastic surgeon right after he diagnosed her with breast cancer. She had cancer in only one of her breasts; however, since implants were available, her surgeon recommended that she have both breasts removed. According to both her oncologist and her plastic surgeon, this surgery would prevent the spread of cancer in her healthy breast while producing a better "cosmetic result." (Without the insertion of two implants, Kate would have been "lopsided.") Believing her doctors knew best, Kate went along with their recommendation and had a bilateral mastectomy and skin expanders placed in her chest wall, which were later replaced with two implants.

Kate and a few other women I interviewed wondered if they would have opted to undergo breast reconstruction if they had been given more time to think about this decision. In Kate's case, she was asked to decide whether or not she wanted reconstructive surgery on the same day she was diagnosed with breast cancer. In hindsight, she believed that she was "more or less in a state of shock" and could not make a sound choice at that time. Brenda, too, was encouraged by her physician to make a decision about receiving breast implants soon after she was told she had cancer. Describing the circumstances under which she decided to have implants, Brenda illustrates how this choice was constrained by the medical context that shaped it:

> [After my diagnosis], I was introduced to the plastic surgeon who was brought in to give me information on the reconstructive procedure. Now, when these doctors explain this surgery to you, you do not necessarily understand it. You don't understand it, your spouse doesn't understand it. . . . I am now so much against doctors encouraging this surgery because I was not mentally all there at that point to make such a decision. Not only was I not mentally correct to make it, but I did not understand what the plastic surgeon was saying to me and the terms he was using. I just went along with it.

Brenda eventually learned that reconstructive surgery involving breast implants can be a long, drawn-out process involving months of physician visits and physical pain. Because women who undergo radical mastectomies are left with no breast tissue, their skin needs to be expanded before an implant can be properly inserted. An expander is placed underneath the skin where the mastectomy is performed and over the course of several weeks or months is slowly filled with saline solution. Once the skin is sufficiently stretched out, the expander is removed, and an implant is inserted. In hindsight, Brenda was certain she would not have opted to receive implants if she had been fully aware of the time and pain involved. Moreover, she explained, "There became a point in time [while I was going through with the procedure] when I knew that I probably could have put the cancer behind me faster, but this procedure keeps it very much alive—the continuance, it goes on for such a length of time. It is such a time-consuming thing. It takes over your life, basically."

Physicians describe good candidates for breast reconstruction following a mastectomy as being "psychologically stable . . . not doing it for ulterior motives—such as a fear that they're going to lose their spouse unless they go through with it or any reason other than simply wanting to restore their appearance or just be more comfortable in clothes."[44] Iris Young argues that statements such as this, along with the popular literature about breast loss, which is "full of stories of the selfless and magnanimous men who stand by their women, insisting that they love her and not her breasts," are based on a male-centered view of women's emotional trauma from breast loss.[45] Indeed, none of the ten women I spoke with who had their breasts reconstructed with implants following a mastectomy felt that their spouses or lovers had pressured them into restoring their appearances.[46] Nevertheless, they were confronted with other emotional challenges linked to the loss of their breasts.

By definition, "reconstructive" surgery involving breast implants is "medically necessary." Such a label perpetuates the idea that breast reconstruction is an integral part of the cancer recovery process, while assuming that the primary concern of all women who are about to undergo mastectomies is their physical appearance. Within cultural and medical contexts that define women by their bodily attributes, women who are faced with the loss of their breasts are perceived as having only two alternatives: either wearing an uncomfortable exterior prosthesis or restoring their "disfigured" and "unfeminine" appearances back to "normal" by undergoing breast reconstruction. Georgine, a woman who had implants to enlarge the size of her breasts commented, "I have never had cancer. I have never been in that situation. But, I guess a woman who has cancer really has no choice [about undergoing breast reconstruction]. I mean, for me, [implantation] was my choice. I guess that is the difference." Some women perceive those who had breast implants for "cosmetic" reasons as having little choice in the matter. Suzanne, who had implants following a mastectomy, explained, "You know, versus passing judgment on women [who had implants to enlarge their breasts], I believe that those women need more compassion than the women, like myself, who had breast cancer. Women who had implants [for cosmetic reasons] were so disconnected from their bodies that they had surgery to restructure them. My heart goes out to those women who just blindly go on and do that."

While the women I interviewed who had implants for both reconstructive and cosmetic purposes were not "blindly" duped by the cultural image of ideal female attractiveness, they also did not perceive themselves as "active agents" who chose to undergo plastic surgery in order to take hold of their lives. The descriptions women provided of their reasons for seeking implants suggest that although they participated in the medicalization of femininity by undergoing surgery to reshape or reconstruct their breasts, this participation had more to do with the specific nature of their subordination than their capacity to take action over their life circumstances. In particular, many women who had implants for "cosmetic" reasons explained that the nature of their interpersonal relationships shaped their decision to seek breast implants. Their husbands, peers, and parents had internalized prevailing cultural assumptions that a woman's primary asset is her physical appearance, and that in order for her to be valued, she must adhere to a narrowly defined cultural image of female attractiveness. For these women, the decision to receive breast implants had more to do with succumbing to interpersonal pressure than with taking action to overcome resistance.

Women's descriptions of their interactions with plastic surgeons also suggest that the decision to reshape one's body is less a reflection of "agency" than it is a manifestation of the specific nature of women's subordination. Just as women's partners, family members, and friends had internalized the cultural assumption that a woman's self-worth is intrinsically linked to her appearance, so, too, did their plastic surgeons. These physicians convinced many women that they would be "better off" with bodies that resembled a cultural ideal of female beauty, characterized by large breasts. Women I interviewed who simply wanted their surgeons to "lift" their sagging breast tissue, which had resulted from nursing or bodily changes after their pregnancies, were told that breast augmentation with implants would be a simple and safe procedure that would make them look "beautiful."

Several of the women I interviewed who received implants following a mastectomy also explained that their physicians influenced their decision to undergo surgery with breast implants. These women reported that their doctors began talking about the replacement of their real breast(s) with one(s) made of silicone immediately after they had been diagnosed with breast cancer. Although these women were initially comforted by their decision to undergo reconstructive surgery, after learning that breast implants could cause serious health problems, they began to question the larger cultural context that shaped their reasons for going through with this procedure. Many of them came to understand that their reasons for wanting to restore their bodies back to normalcy were linked to a society in which femininity is deeply connected to women's physical appearance. They believed that if they had been given the opportunity to reflect on their experiences with loss and grief, and if they had been fully aware of the pain, discomfort, and possible side effects associated with breast implantation, they would not have gone through with this surgery.

4

False Expectations
An Ironic Twist on "Before and After"

omen who are considering breast implants are
often handed binders filled with glossy pages of
photos of women's breasts. To preserve their
anonymity, the heads of the women in the pictures have
been lopped off—so that what remains are pages upon pages
of breasts, always two photos side by side: The image on the
left is "before" implantation, and the one on the right is "after" the procedure. Sometimes there is only a slight difference between the two photos: The two breasts on the right
are slightly rounder and larger than the ones on the left. In
other cases, the difference is quite drastic: The image on the
left shows the asymmetry of a woman's body after a radical
mastectomy—a slightly concave and scarred chest wall adjacent to one breast. The image on the right displays the
same body after reconstruction; a scarred mound has replaced the concave chest wall. In some of these images there
is no nipple. In other pictures, a nipple has been tattooed
onto the mound resembling a breast.

Two of the women I interviewed mentioned that after
seeing such photos, they asked their surgeons if they could
speak to women who had already received implants, perhaps
wanting to put faces, or identities, to the headless, dismem-
bered bodies displayed across the pages in those black binders. Speaking to actual women about their experiences with
implants could confirm the positive results conveyed by the

photos. Some surgeons have lists of women willing to share these experiences. Jenna, for example, remembered: "I asked [the plastic surgeon] for a couple of phone numbers of women who had had breast implants. I wanted to see what they say. And, when I called these women, they were really thrilled. They said that their husbands thought that they were beautiful. It just all sounded too good to be true."

In Paula's case, her plastic surgeon introduced her to one of his patients who had recently undergone breast reconstruction with an implant. She explained, "Right there in the plastic surgeon's office, he had another woman [who had just received a breast implant]. He said, 'I just did this woman. Let me have you talk to her.' So she came in and we revealed ourselves [showed their breasts] to each other, and I really liked the work he had done on her. And so, I said, 'Okay, I will have you do the operation.'"

Although the women I interviewed were impressed with before-and-after photographs and conversations they had with their surgeons' former patients, many explained that they remained apprehensive about the procedure. Feeling that the results they were viewing were simply "too good to be true," many asked their surgeons about any short- or long-term risks associated with implants. Most were told that breast implants are "perfectly safe."

In examining women's lives after receiving implants, I call into question Kathy Davis's analysis of women's experiences with cosmetic surgery.[1] The women Davis interviewed who had their breasts enlarged with implants reported that they were misinformed of the risks associated with this procedure prior to undergoing it. In this respect, Davis's sample is similar to my own.[2] However, while Davis reports that women who undergo cosmetic surgery are unaware of the potential dangers associated breast implants, she maintains the view that these women are fully aware of the cultural context that shapes their decision to enlarge their breasts. In other words, women who undergo cosmetic surgery understand that the media and other social institutions construct a false ideal of feminine beauty while perpetuating a homogenous representation of the female body. Davis thus argues that women are not passive victims of an oppressive, patriarchal society that forces them into conformity. Rather, women are agents, "who creatively and knowledgeably negotiate their lives, even under circumstances which are not of their own making."[3]

A woman's decision to undergo cosmetic surgery, therefore, is not a simple one but is fraught with conflict and deliberation. To verify the emphasis she places on women's agency over structural influences in women's decision-making process, Davis includes in her analysis follow-up interviews with twelve women who had undergone breast augmentation. She interviewed these women prior to surgery, immediately after it, and one year later in order to understand how women, in hindsight, make sense of their decision to reshape their bodies. Using the experiences of these women, she addresses the following questions: "How do [women] regard [their decision to undergo cosmetic surgery] in the light of the outcome of the operation? Are they still convinced that cosmetic surgery has enabled them to take control over their lives? Do they continue to regard it as their best option under the circumstances or do they feel that they have been had and that cosmetic surgery is anything but a choice?"[4] Davis found that her respondents, even a year after they had had their surgeries, continued to consider their cosmetic surgery as a "choice in a context where they had no other recourse."[5] In other words, aware that Western culture is fraught with myths about femininity and female attractiveness, these women continued to believe that, given their circumstances, they had made the best choice possible to alleviate their own personal suffering.

Davis reports that, for the most part, the women she interviewed were quite satisfied with the outcomes of their surgeries: "Some were unreservedly enthusiastic, describing their breasts as 'really beautiful,' or 'just gorgeous.' Others were more reticent, yet still pleased ('it is much better than I had expected,' 'one hundred percent better than it was'). They continually contrasted their previous suffering with examples which illustrated how improved their lives had become."[6] She found that even women who experienced unexpected hardening, pain, and discomfort after their surgeries were nevertheless glad that they had made the choice to have breast implants. In fact, she spoke with only two women who had experienced the severe implant-related health problems and complications that over half of the women in my sample of forty were experiencing. Davis explains her negative cases as exceptions or "dramatic stories," differing from the positive accounts told by the greater proportion of her sample. In my study, the tables are turned—Davis's negative, or exceptional, cases reflect the situation found in over half of my cases. Indeed, my recruitment strategy may have elicited more responses from women who had negative experiences with breast implants than from women who were satisfied with the outcome of their surgeries.[7] But, while my sample may (or may not) represent the experiences of the majority of women who have breast implants, it nevertheless provides the opportunity to explore, theoretically, how some women come to view their decision to seek breast implants several (for some women, more than twenty) years after the fact.

Experiencing a New Body

When I asked women how they felt about their new bodies after surgery, half of the women I interviewed were "thrilled" with their new breasts: Clothing fit them better, and they felt more confident both socially and sexually. In this way, my findings resonate with those presented in Davis's analysis.[8] According to the majority of women Davis interviewed and some of the women I spoke with, receiving breast implants provided a way to renegotiate their identities, to reconceptualize their bodies in relation to a new sense of self. For example, Joyce, who had undergone breast augmentation over ten years ago, recalled, "After I had the surgery, for the first time in my life, I really felt like I was a whole person, like everybody else. I had self-confidence and was able to wear anything I wanted. I didn't feel threatened." Mona, who had her breast implants in 1975, explained, "Having implants just made me feel a little more—not so vulnerable. . . . Looking back at pictures when I was eighteen, my shoulders were hunched over to cover up my body because I felt so ashamed."

Similarly, Eve described how having implants improved her self-esteem: "[After receiving the implants] it was almost like I stood up straighter, I walked straighter and it just gave me a little more self-esteem. I didn't go into hysterics trying to find a bathing suit or I didn't worry about wearing baggy clothes so nobody could see. . . . Initially I was pretty ecstatic. I don't know how to describe it—proud." Once entrapped in bodies that seemed "different" and "abnormal," these women saw their decision to receive breast implants as a liberating experience. Plastic surgery provided them with the opportunity to move through life with more confidence and pride. It enabled them to transform their identities. For some women, their newfound self-assurance after receiving breast implants transcended their social and sexual lives. Sarah explained, "Well, having implants, kind of changed—I don't want to say behavior, but it kind of changed the way I acted with other people. I felt more confident about myself. And plus, if I had a relationship, it was a little bit easier to expose myself."

The women I spoke with who had such positive experiences after they had undergone their surgeries explained that they perceived their implants as parts of their own bodies. Feeling less self-conscious about their appearances and more self-confident about themselves, these women conceptually incorporated their new breasts into their sense of self or being. Women who had reconstructive surgery with implants after mastectomies felt similarly. Suzanne, who had a bilateral mastectomy, referred to her new breasts after implantation as her "new girls." She explained that she "really embraced [the implants], taking them into [her] body" as if they truly were a part of her self.

Despite these positive responses, twenty of the forty women I interviewed experienced mixed emotions, or a sense of inner conflict, after receiving breast implants. In fact, contrary to Davis's findings, the majority of the women I interviewed were angry, explicitly stating that they felt pressured into putting something into their bodies to fulfill a societal standard of femininity or sexuality.[9] For instance, Jenna admitted that after receiving implants in 1989 she felt more "sexually confident." She also explained that her new breast size was a convenience— especially in the summertime since "they don't make bathing suits for people with size 'A' breasts and size 10 hips." But, at the same time, Jenna described feeling a strange "split" in attitude about having the implants: "I didn't feel good about feeling more sexual with the implants. . . . I was really angry inside that I had had to put plastic bags filled with chemicals in my body in order for me to feel like I could do the Hoochie Koo on Saturday nights. . . . I felt a lot of shame about what I had done. I didn't wear tight clothes, I didn't wear low-cut things, I didn't want my children to find out."

Whereas Jenna directed her anger about "what [she] had done" toward herself, others directed these feelings outward. For instance, Leslie felt hostility toward her surgeon after her operation: "When I first got the implants, I was very angry at the surgeon. I used to be this small, little, petite person in stature and I could wear these cutesy little things and I mean—that was a part of who I was. I mean, I don't think I realized how much a wardrobe is actually a statement about yourself. . . . It was like [the surgeon] didn't tell me that this was going to happen. That part of me, having to re–figure out a new wardrobe and develop into a

new person. I remember distinctly feeling angry and lost—not knowing who this person was." And Ann, who has had her implants for
twenty-three years now, vividly remembered the feelings she experienced during her operation, directing her anger at yet another source.
She recalled, "I was awake for the surgery and remembered seeing my
reflection in the light and sort of seeing my body cut open. It was very
bizarre because they put the screen in front of you so you don't see what
is going on, but I am watching the surgery from above me. Then, as
soon as it was done, I sat up and felt this well of anger. Like, look what
they had done to me, *they* collectively—the collective world, the whole
shebang—that *they* had to just cut up my body and stick these things in
me." As Ann watched her surgeon cut open her body and insert two
shiny, silicone-filled plastic bags, she became acutely aware of her feeling that her decision to be on the operating table was not entirely her
own—*society* was at fault for making her feel unimportant without larger
breasts.

These women received breast implants in the hope of improving
their self-esteem and poor sense of body-image. However, unlike those
women who were pleased with their new bodies after they had received
breast implants, about half of the women I spoke with were unaware of
the difficulties involved in renegotiating their new bodies with their
sense of self. These women were unprepared to deal with the emotional ramifications of their bodily transformations. Ann, for instance,
explained that she eventually overcame the initial anger she experienced
after her surgery, and was left with a strange curiosity about having a
different body, "this sexy, attractive body." At the same time, however,
she explained that she always felt like she "was faking it"—presenting
herself as someone who she really was not. Her feeling of separation
from body and self intensified anytime she met a man who was attracted
to her. The thought that someday she was going to have to tell a potential lover about her breast implants was unbearable: "I was afraid of
being found out. . . . My implants were my deep dark secret." Some of
the women I interviewed chose not to divulge this secret to their partners. Sarah had her surgery before she was married, not telling her husband that she had implants until she became concerned that she was
experiencing adverse health effects from the devices.

The secrecy around having breast implants is linked to the broader
issue of how women, in general, respond to societal standards of femininity and female attractiveness. Displeased with the way they naturally

appear, women often feel embarrassed and ashamed about taking part in beauty practices in order to adhere to cultural ideals of female bodily perfection and appearance. After admitting to her own personal suffering around ideas of female beauty and confessing to her own beauty secret (electrolysis treatment for hair removal), the feminist scholar Wendy Chapkis describes all women as

> foreigners attempting to assimilate into a hostile culture, our bodies continually threatening to betray our difference. Each of us who seeks the rights of citizenship through acceptable femininity shares a secret with all who attempt to pass: My undisguised self is unacceptable, I am not what I seem. To successfully pass is to be momentarily wrapped in the protective cover of conformity. To fail is to experience the vulnerability of the outsider.
>
> Despite the fact that each woman knows her own belabored transformation from female to feminine is artificial, she harbors the secret conviction that it should be effortless. A "real woman" would be naturally feminine while she is only in disguise. To the uninitiated—men—the image must maintain its mystery, hence the tools of transformation are to be hidden away as carefully as the "flaws" they are used to remedy.[10]

While some women adjusted to their new identities with ease, embracing their breast implants as if they were a part of their own bodies, others experienced inner conflict, a feeling of separation between body and self. Finding their "real" bodies unacceptable, they have put on a disguise—new breasts. Even though they now appeared "natural" and "feminine," they were uncomfortably disconnected from their true selves. These women were left viewing themselves as fakes and frauds, afraid of being found out.

Ironically, while women receive implants in an effort to conform to societal ideas about femininity, some felt uncomfortably obvious and *more* self-conscious about their bodies *after* receiving implants than before. This is another finding that diverges from the results presented in Davis's research.[11] While nearly all of the women Davis interviewed were happy with their cosmetic surgeries, some of the women I interviewed felt more like sex objects with their new bodies. Hillary, for instance, wore bulky sweaters or baggy T-shirts to hide her new breasts, because she was so embarrassed about them. Similarly, Lorraine explained that after she received breast implants, her new breasts made her feel like she was on display: "I felt very obvious. I don't feel like they are me, you know? I have always carried that." Lorraine explained how these feelings affected her social life: "When I was single and dated fellows, I wouldn't dance close. I was always afraid that you could tell by getting up close, holding somebody close, or anything that gets that way. If nothing else, getting implants was the best birth control—sex shut down." Even though the prevailing belief in American culture is that women with larger breasts are expected to be more sexual and alluring, many women, like Lorraine, avoided potential sexual encounters in an effort to keep their implants a secret.

In Christine's case, she mistakenly believed that her breast implants would save her marriage and improve her sex life with her husband, who no longer found her attractive. About a year after her surgery, she and her husband were divorced. When she entered the dating scene again, she began to believe that men were attracted to her body rather than her personality: "I wonder how my life would have been different if I hadn't attracted men based on my boobs rather than on who I was." Christine's statement again reveals a disjunction, or split, between body and self. Her breast implants changed her outward appearance, while concealing her true identity.

Nina also felt self-conscious after she had her breasts enlarged, always wondering how people perceived her: "I felt out of proportion. I felt like I was way too top-heavy and became very focused on the reaction and response of whether I looked normal or not. I was very concerned about what other people thought of me. After a while, I began to—I guess I want to say 'owned' the body image and thought the implants made me more sensual and sexually desirable."

Like Nina, some women eventually accepted their implants as a part of their own bodies and incorporated their new breasts into their sense of self. For Sheila, however, fifteen years passed before she began to feel as though her breasts were her own: "I really didn't think of [my breasts] as mine. I thought of them as a cosmetic thing that I did." When I asked Sheila what made her recently feel more connected to her implants, she explained, "I guess it was maturity, getting older and, you know, accepting that I [had gotten the implants], accepting the reasons why I did it, and I made it okay." Implicit in Sheila's explanation are elements of self-blame and forgiveness. For fifteen years following her surgery, Sheila was unable to fully comprehend the larger context that shaped her reasons for receiving implants. She had not allowed herself to feel connected with her implants, because she felt that she had done something "cosmetic" and superficial. In fact, unlike many women, Sheila was quite open about having breast implants, telling women who admired her figure, "Well, you can do this too!" Only in hindsight did Sheila realize that her reasons for seeking implants were linked to pressure from her ex-husband (who was a "boob man"), and a poor sense of who she was in relation to her body. As she grew older, she could look back on her past self and understand the context that perpetuated her negative self-image. This understanding allowed her to reconceptualize her reasons for seeking implants as not just something she had done for "cosmetic" reasons, but as something she felt at the time she had to do under specific circumstances.

For a few women, the sense of feeling separated or detached from their bodies after implantation was a more gradual experience. Not until two years after she had her surgery did Beth begin to question why she had decided to have her breasts enlarged. She explained that immediately after her surgery, "my self-esteem was very high, I felt beautiful, I felt feminine, I had breasts—it was wonderful. Clothes looked great on me, they were beautiful to look at, it was very aesthetically pleasing for me." However, she said that two years after she had the procedure, "I started looking at myself again and started changing. . . . I began to feel separate from the implants themselves. They weren't a part of me—they weren't part of my body, it was an invasion, a manmade thing that probably shouldn't have been put in my body. . . . Although getting the implants was a decision that was made over a year's time, it all seemed too hasty. I started regretting what I had done."

Davis argues that receiving cosmetic surgery, for many women, is perceived as an "empowering" or "liberating" experience. Surgery provides women who feel trapped inside a body that does not fit their sense of self with a way to renegotiate their identity.[12] This interpretation fits with half of the experiences reported to me by the women I interviewed. The experiences of the other half of my respondents indicate that this transformation in self after receiving breast implants is not always met with ease, but often with confusion and anger. These women came to view their altered outward appearances as a disjunction from self, rather than as a unification of body and identity. Many blamed their doctors, themselves, and the larger society for perpetuating ideals about femininity and female bodies that diverged from the shapes of their own bodies. Many felt embarrassed and ashamed about having surgically altered their bodies. They did not carry their heads high and chests up, but tried to conceal their new bodies with bulky clothing and attempted to keep their implants a secret from potential lovers.

The Progression of Symptoms and the Loss of Self

Not only were some women dismayed that their breast implants failed to improve their social and sexual lives, but to make matters worse, thirty-five of the forty women interviewed reported having experienced complications directly related to their implants, such as deflation or ruptures leading to multiple replacement surgeries and the formation of scar tissue around the implants. Moreover, thirty-four of the forty women I interviewed believe they are now experiencing physical symptoms associated with their implants. These symptoms include joint pain, hair loss, infertility problems, chronic infections, headaches, chronic fatigue, chronic allergies, chronic fever and sore throats, asthma, difficulty swallowing, spontaneous bruising, loss of cognitive functioning, dry membranes (including eyes, mouth, and vaginal area), disorientation or dizziness, irregular menses, speech difficulties, rashes, lumps in breast, numbness, hot flashes, respiratory problems, dental problems, loss of sex drive, memory loss, abdominal pain, burning in chest area, sleep disturbances, visual disturbances, sudden weight gain, photosensitivity, chest pain, and loss of nipple sensation. Only five out of the forty women I spoke with reported no symptoms and no implant-related complications.

Twenty-five of the women I interviewed were also diagnosed with one or more of the following diseases after they received their implants: rheumatoid arthritis, fibromyalgia, irritable bowel syndrome, chronic fatigue syndrome, lupus, Sjögren's syndrome, scleroderma, Reynaud's disease, cancer, and peripheral neuropathy. Seven women out of the forty interviewed had children after receiving breast implants. Four of these women reported that their children are also experiencing health effects believed to be related to migrating silicone, including digestive problems, aching joints, chronic fatigue, rashes, and cognitive difficulties.

The differences between the quality of life these women had before they received breast implants and after they began to experience implant-related health problems cast an ironic twist on the "before and after" comparisons presented to them in the glossy pages of plastic surgery binders before their surgeries. A device intended to improve women's bodily appearance, as well as their social and sexual lives, has left many women disabled and disfigured. Breast implants initially may have given these women the appearance (and for some, the identity) they had always wanted, but at a cost they would never have imagined. Well over half of the women I interviewed suffered extreme losses because their implant-related illnesses prevented them from participating in normal, daily-life activities. A quarter of my respondents, for instance, had lost their jobs and their future earning potential because they were too sick to work. Nearly 20 percent of the women I spoke with reported that they could no longer socialize because they tired easily or became disoriented whenever they left their homes. And, 25 percent of the women I interviewed reported experiencing marital problems stemming from their inability to meet their husbands' sexual and social needs. Christine's story particularly illuminates the irony of "before and after."

"A Chemically Toxic Person": Christine's Story

I conducted my interview with Christine in her home in a quiet suburb outside of San Francisco. She has her own house; however, about a year prior to our meeting, she took in two boarders to help with the mortgage. Because the house has only two bedrooms, now both occupied by these tenants, Christine has moved most of her belongings into the living room. As we entered into this room, I noticed a stack of books in boxes appearing half-unpacked. Clothing was scattered about, and to my left was a makeshift bed—a sofa with a sheet and blanket neatly tucked into the cushions and a pillow at one end. I sensed that Christine was somewhat embarrassed by the clutter as she rushed me through the room and into a small den off the kitchen. As we passed through, she explained, "I moved my things in the living room, but really it doesn't matter where my bed is since I don't sleep anyway."

I knew the meaning implicit in Christine's words. By the time I met with her, I had already interviewed about thirty women for my research—enough to know that insomnia is a common symptom experienced by women who have received breast implants. Christine's appearance, that is, her ashen complexion, droopy, tired eyes, and the red, blotchy rash covering her cheeks, were also familiar indicators—probably early signs of lupus or some other autoimmune disease. Christine resembled many of the women I had already met during the course of my research, women who had once been active and energetic, but were now ill, chronically fatigued, and suffering from persistent pain.[13] All of these women believe that their decline in health is related to a decision they ironically had made to improve their lives—their decision to seek breast implants.

Christine and I sat on a couch, legs tilted inward so that we were facing each other. Before Christine began her story, she asked if I would mind if she stretched her legs. "Of course, I don't mind," I responded. As she tucked a couple of pillows between her back and the arm of the sofa and raised her legs on the middle cushion in between us to make herself comfortable, she began to tell me about her life before her health problems began.

Christine was always a hard worker. By the time she was eighteen years old, she had become trained as a dental hygienist and then put herself through college as well as a doctoral program in chiropractics, by working part-time in a dentist's office. After she finished her schooling in 1987, she continued with this job in order to support herself while she was starting up a new practice. Christine also had a busy social life—downhill skiing, hiking, and mountain climbing were just a few of her pastimes. Another one of Christine's favorite pursuits was flying. Before she started graduate school, she had managed to become an aerobatic pilot, striving to defy all odds by wing-walking on airplanes.

While she was telling me about this life, Christine scrambled up from her seat, disappeared for a moment, and returned with a few photographs. I took a look. One of the pictures, which had been taken about three years ago, was of the exterior of her old office when she was a chiropractor. Her practice was located in a seaside village. The office itself was a shingle-covered, solar-heated dome, and a plaque with her name engraved on it was tacked up on the right of the door. Another picture, taken at around the same time, was of a beautiful woman, with dark eyes and a vibrant smile. She was wearing a white lab coat. The woman looked vaguely familiar, but only upon closer examination did I realize that she was Christine. Showing me this photo, she explained to me, "Back then I was a real gregarious person . . . who loved to have an audience." Although I did not ask Christine why she showed me these photos, I sensed that she did so because she was not sure I would believe her own description of herself without some solid evidence of her past life. Her action, ironically, was similar to the actions of plastic surgeons—in order to convince their patients that their lives will be "different" after their cosmetic surgeries, they, too, present them with solid evidence—before-and-after photos. I have to admit that imagining the woman in the picture as an energetic, outgoing individual who took part in athletic activities and daredevil stunts on airplanes was easy. Imagining the woman who now sat by my side as possessing these characteristics was much more difficult.

Christine had received implants in 1970, at the age of twenty-nine. About four years afterwards, she began to experience a series of peculiar, vague symptoms: Her memory became fuzzy, she began to experience a strange tingling in her mouth and swelling of her tongue every time she drank wine or other alcoholic beverages, and a strange dark spot had appeared on her labia, which was undiagnosed.[14] A few years later, she began experiencing other symptoms, such as aching joints and stomach irritability. By the mid-1980s, while Christine was completing her doctoral degree, she was diagnosed with irritable bowel syndrome. At this time, she also developed more serious problems: "I had problems with my eyes; I had problems with high blood pressure; I hemorrhaged for a few weeks straight—blood vessels would break. . . . I began to have trouble with reading comprehension and developed headaches so bad that I had to stop flying because they would intensify with the change in altitude." Concerned about these health problems, Christine took a sample of her blood to one of her instructors to look at under a microscope. Upon his examination, he discovered some unusual, atypical, white blood cells and explained to Christine that they were indicative of lupus. Despite these findings, the instructor reassured Christine that her blood was probably drawn incorrectly, which would distort the cells and give false results. With this explanation, Christine decided not to worry and began to attribute all of her strange symptoms to stress. She simply figured that the long hours she was putting in at school and at her part-time job as a hygienist were taking a toll on her health. Attempting to dismiss her symptoms as minor inconveniences, she continued on with her life.

By 1989, Christine had completed her schooling and was continuing to work part-time as a dental hygienist. During this year, she began to develop other problems. Now appearing on her face was a strange, blotchy rash that, according to several dermatologists she had visited, was undiagnosable as well as incurable. As the rash worsened, Christine's employer increasingly complained about her appearance, saying that he did not like the way her face looked and that he felt uncomfortable with her working closely with his patients. Although she had been working for this dentist for fifteen years, he fired her two weeks before Christmas.

In 1990, Christine managed to find another part-time job as a dental hygienist but began to notice that she was becoming increasingly fatigued during the days. She could barely get out of bed some mornings and was missing days of work. At her own practice, she could no longer carry on a full day's work without napping during her lunch and coffee breaks. One day she even fell asleep while working on a patient.

Despite all of her symptoms, Christine refused to believe that she had a serious health problem. She went into what she refers to as her "period of denial," believing that her symptoms were the result of "being so active": "I decided that whenever I didn't feel well, it was because I was doing too much." In hindsight, not only does Christine believe that she was fooling herself into believing that she was healthy, but she also was hiding her symptoms from her employer: "It just got to a point where I was learning how to lie really well for the first time in my life because I had to in order to keep my job." Eventually, she could no longer hide her chronic fatigue and, once again, lost her job. In total, since 1989, she has been fired from twelve different positions due to her health problems. She explained:

> By midday I looked like somebody ran over me with a truck. I was that fatigued. You know, I would carry on the acts, so to speak, for the morning, but the afternoon would come around, and I would have a lot more troubles. And, you know, most dentists—they want somebody who is real cheerful. And, I mean, when you are—it's a people's business and they need to have somebody that is not just—it doesn't matter if you can do a good job cleaning teeth—you have to do PR work, too, really. And, I can understand that. Frankly, if I was a dentist, I wouldn't have wanted me to work for him or her.

Fortunately, Christine had enough money saved to support herself for a while after she became unemployed. Still feeling tired and achy practically every minute of each day, in 1992, she decided that she could use a vacation and rented a cabin in the mountains with a group of her friends. She purchased a season's ski pass, thinking to herself, "Okay, now I am really going to get healthy by skiing and getting in shape." When she got to the slopes, however, she was dismayed to find that she could ski only one to three hours a day before she would have to return to the cabin and collapse on her bed from fatigue. She was used to skiing eight-hour days. At that point, Christine knew that "something was really, really wrong."

In addition to her physical problems, when Christine returned home from her vacation, she developed cognitive difficulties: "I couldn't dial the phone anymore because if I looked at the phone number, I couldn't remember it from the page long enough to get it in the phone. I couldn't think of words when I—I had aphasia to the point where I couldn't talk without constantly stopping and then I would have to try to think of another word in its place. And—that was very difficult for me because I had always considered myself such a bright person."

Not until Christine joined a support group for women with silicone breast implants did she connect her symptoms to her implants. In 1993, she had ex-plantation surgery and, since then, has regained some of her cognitive functioning; although she still, on occasion, has difficulties reading and writing. Despite having her implants removed, Christine's physical problems persist. She has had to give up her practice and is now living on a limited income from her disability insurance.

As Christine sat next to me on the couch in her small den off the kitchen, she gazed with tearful eyes at the photos lying on the coffee table between us. One was of her old practice, and the other of herself in a lab coat taken just a few years ago. Still looking at the pictures, she commented, "I don't know who I am anymore, I really have changed so much. I am not the person I used to be. And it is like—you start thinking to yourself, 'I used to do this, I used to do that; I used to love this, I used to love that; I used to feel this way. . . .' Now, I just see myself as a chemically toxic person."

Christine's case sounds like an exceptionally dramatic one. But, in fact, it is not. In interview after interview, I heard women's stories: the pain and the suffering, the secrecy, denial and self-blame, and the loss of self—the feeling of not knowing who this person is inside this sick and tired body. This loss of identity took on different meanings for different women. For some, the most difficult part about becoming ill was having to give up their careers, their income, and earning potential. Many of the women I interviewed had once satisfying jobs that gave them self-respect and enabled them to be self-supporting. Other women described the loss of identity in terms of their inability to function as wives and mothers.

Secrecy and Denial

Christine's attempts at hiding her illness are similar to other women's accounts of secrecy. Brenda, for example, was suffering from memory loss, chronic fatigue, arthritis, and connective-tissue disease—all of which she attributed to the breast implants she had after her mastectomy in 1986. Like Christine, the progression of Brenda's symptoms was gradual. She initially attributed her aching joints and fatigue to her age. At fifty-one years old, she thought that perhaps she was supposed to be suffering from some of these symptoms.[15] But not only did these health problems worsen, new ones emerged: Her memory started to fail, and she developed connective-tissue disease that affected her gums, causing her to lose all of her teeth. At this point, Brenda really thought she was "going crazy." Speaking for other women who similarly have received implants, she explained, "Not every woman who has implants has been diagnosed with a disease. And, if they are menopausal, and perhaps have had their breasts removed, and have all of these problems, they just get the feeling that they are just plain going crazy. They are isolated, they are alone, they are afraid. And you start to remove yourself from the rest of society because you can't keep up. And you start hiding things. And you start kidding yourself, basically, in the hopes of being part of the everyday norm." Brenda further explained that because many women with implants appear healthy, friends and family frequently tell them, "Hey, you are not looking all that bad, you look pretty good." In Brenda's case, these words reinforced her denial of her own illness: "You start participating in looking good. This keeps the secret going."

For other women, the discrepancy between their outward appearances and the societal perception of what sick people should look like led their physicians to minimize and dismiss their symptoms. For instance, Joyce visited a rheumatologist because, for months, she had been experiencing aching joints and "sleeping half to three quarters of the day." Despite these symptoms, the doctor took one look at Joyce and said, "You have a great tan, you look great—what are you so worried about?" Since by all outward appearances Joyce was "healthy" and "looked great," her doctor saw no reason to search for a physical explanation for her reported symptoms; instead, she told Joyce, "I think that [your problem] is psychological. I suggest you have a psychiatric evaluation." After hearing this comment, Joyce began to think that perhaps her problem really was "all in [her] head." Taking her doctor's advice, she went to visit a psychiatrist, who misdiagnosed her as manic-depressive and put her on a variety of drugs that made her extremely sick and depressed. After months of suffering from the side effects of these drugs and her continued aching joints and fatigue, Joyce finally decided to visit a doctor who specialized in manic depression. After several visits, he told her that she definitely did not have this psychiatric disorder and recommended that she see different doctors about her physical symptoms.

Joyce's case demonstrates the extent to which an individual's outward appearance can be inconsistent with his or her physical complaints, and how such a discrepancy can perpetuate self-doubt and denial among those who are truly sick. Even though Joyce felt physically sick, she looked healthy. This incongruity led her doctors to invalidate her belief that something was physically wrong with her, and reinforce the notion that her problems were psychological.[16]

Job Loss

In many ways, Christine's story is also similar to Nina's. Nina is a single thirty-eight-year-old woman who has never been married and presently lives in a small apartment with her young son. Like so many women who are experiencing implant-related symptoms, the gradual deterioration of Nina's health sent her into a tailspin of job loss, unemployment, and, in Nina's case, temporary homelessness. Like others whom I interviewed, Nina suffers from chronic fatigue, respiratory problems, hair loss, constant infections, dry membranes and cognitive difficulties that impede her ability to work. Her only income now comes from the disability checks she receives once a month. Nina's description of an episode during a day at her part-time job at a bank is particularly notable: "I was trying to count cash. And, I remember I felt like my brain was frying. I was counting the money and all of a sudden—it was like imagining what it would feel like to have something in your body short-circuit. It just felt like my whole nervous system fried and I could actually hear it sizzle. And then, I could barely even count the money. It was the most bizarre experience. And, for somebody, like myself, who had been through college—I just couldn't count the cash." Like many women who tried to hide their health problems from their employers, Nina explained, "looking good at all costs was the exterior philosophy I was living."[17] Eventually losing her job, Nina saw no alternative but to apply for disability insurance from the government since she was too incapacitated to work. However, the long, tedious, bureaucratic process of applying and being accepted for financial aid forced Nina to give up her apartment and temporarily move into a homeless shelter with her son.

Twenty-five percent of the women I interviewed are now receiving monthly payments from the government because they have been diagnosed with an implant-related illness that prevents them from participating in the workforce. Sheila, for instance, had to give up her lucrative career in retail because she had developed chronic fatigue syndrome and a number of other autoimmune-related symptoms after receiving breast implants twenty years ago. She explained, "I wanted a full life. I had been very successful in my job. . . . I made an incredible living. I never had to worry about money. After my divorce I could financially take care of the kids. There was never 'Oh, you will have to ask your father.' I mean, I really wanted to be a financially and emotionally independent person. I worked really hard to get to that point. And now, I am on disability, and my income is cut by two-thirds. I have had to become dependent. I had to become dependent on family and friends." Other women, who are not receiving disability compensation but still suffer from health effects believed to be implant-related, explained how they, too, have lost their earning potential. Gloria, for example, is a nurse and used to work seven days a week, but is now able to work only part-time because she suffers from chronic fatigue, aches and pains, and other symptoms associated with Sjögren's syndrome and scleroderma.[18] Similarly, Rose used to be a full-time legal secretary and has had to cut down on her hours due to her poor health. She explained, "You know, all my life I thought that if anything happened with my job, I could always wait tables if I had to support myself. And I never—I foolishly never planned for the future because I always thought that I would be healthy. I never dreamed that I would be in the situation I am in now, doing without a TV and things like that because I can't work."

From Wife and Mother to Feeling "Kind of Half-Dead"

Many of the women I spoke with who developed health problems after receiving breast implants say that the worst part of their illness experience is not the physical pain they endure daily but the emotional loss of their sense of identity. Some women described this loss in terms of the transition from being able to support themselves financially to depending on family or the welfare system for economic support. For others, their loss of self was related to their increasing inability to fulfill their roles as housewives or mothers. Jenna, for example, stated:

> My children are upset. They went to the fireworks on the Fourth of July, and I couldn't go because I can barely walk from here to the corner of our street. I just can't do things like that with them anymore. My daughter will say, "I wish you weren't sick," or, "When are you going to get better?" or, "Are you going to die?"—things like that. Some days I can't drive. I have to have help in the house now with cleaning because I can't move my hands to clean because of the pain. And, I can't be involved in my kids' school activities and go on class trips. I haven't been able to do that now in a year. That has been the worse part of it. I don't care that I can't run or exercise anymore. That part I can accept. But, the part that is really hard is not being able to be there for my kids.

Jenna further illustrated how her illness has impacted upon her relationship with her husband, who threatened to leave her because he was unable to cope with her health problems:

> My husband told me that he wasn't getting his needs met. He just expected me to have faith that everything was going to be okay and to get beside my fears and anxieties and still be able to have sex with him and be a functional wife and mother like I had always been. And now, I am just feeling really powerless and trapped because I am sick and I don't know how much sicker I am going to get. And, I can't even fight back anymore because I don't have the energy. I just kind of feel half-dead.

Another similar case is Joyce, who explained how her illness has affected her relationship with her six-year-old son, Adam: "I was probably sleeping half to three-quarters of the day. I was not doing any of my household chores. I had a little boy and, I mean, he would ask me for a glass of water and I would lay there and, honest to God, I could not get up and get him that water. And then I would sit there crying, feeling guilty because I couldn't even give him a glass of water and I would just drag him in on the couch with me and say, 'Stay here with me.' He would lay there for hours sleeping with me." Soon after Joyce received her implants, she became pregnant with Adam. Adam also has developed implant-related symptoms: stomach problems, aching joints, and strange rashes. Joyce's guilt about her inability to perform her tasks as a mother is compounded by her son's illness, which she believes to be directly related to her decision to undergo breast augmentation prior to her pregnancy. Eve, who has an eleven-month-old baby with gastrointestinal difficulties, similarly felt this guilt, stating, "I wonder if I should have even gotten pregnant."

Most of the women I interviewed had experienced some kind of loss or tragedy. Some had lost their jobs. Others had lost their ability to take part in sports or other activities they once had enjoyed, such as jogging, biking, and painting. Women also reported that they were no longer able to socialize. They never felt well enough to go for a walk, go out to lunch, or go shopping with their friends. Some women reported that their health had deteriorated so drastically that their spouses walked out on them because they simply were not emotionally equipped to handle the changes in their wives' daily functioning.

Kathy Davis found in her analysis of women's experiences with cosmetic surgery[19] that her respondents, even a year following their surgeries, continued to perceive their decision to undergo cosmetic surgery as a liberating and empowering experience. They took their lives into their own hands, taking what they decided was the best course of action given their circumstances. But, the respondents (with two exceptions) in Davis's follow-up study did not experience the extent of pain, discomfort, and illness described by the women I interviewed. Do women with implants who experience debilitating autoimmune symptoms feel that they made the right choice given their circumstances? Do they take full responsibility for their choice to receive breast implants? Or, do they feel that perhaps they were not fully aware of the larger social, cultural, political, and economic forces at work when they had made their decision?

Davis reports that her respondents seemed more prepared to accept the cultural context that shapes ideas about femininity and female bodies, but less prepared to accept the medical context in which their decisions were taken. Although many were happy with the outcome of their surgeries, they also had learned that their doctors provided them with misleading information about implant-associated risk, and became considerably more "vocal about their right to receive adequate information and to be treated as competent in making their own decisions."[20] Nevertheless, for the most part, these women maintained that they would probably have undergone breast augmentation even if they had been aware of all the known risks.

In her analysis, Davis distinguishes between two separate contexts that shape women's decisions to seek breast implants, or any other form of cosmetic surgery. The first is a cultural context that conveys assumptions about the ideal female body; the second is a medical context in which "physicians systematically withhold information or downplay the risks of surgery."[21] Her emphasis on agency over structural influence as an explanation of why women undergo cosmetic surgery is supported by her analysis of women's awareness of the "cultural context," yet she pays little attention to women's apparent naiveté of the medical context. As was the case with the women I interviewed, Davis herself found that prior to their surgeries, women were not skeptical of medicine but thought that their doctors were "the next best thing to God himself."[22]

In the following chapter, I argue that medical and cultural contexts are inseparable: Ideas about femininity and female bodies transcend medical discourse and shape the information about the benefits and risks of implants conveyed to women by their plastic surgeons. The women I interviewed have constructed their own political, economic, and sometimes feminist critiques of the breast implant disaster. Their theories about why their government, the medical profession, and implant manufactures failed to warn them of the dangers of breast implants prior to their surgeries suggest that they do indeed perceive themselves as victims of a society that places more value on a woman's physical appearance than her health. So, while I agree that agency plays into women's decisions to receive breast implants, I assert that larger structural and cultural factors are of tantamount importance.

5.

Misinforming Women of Risk

A Medical Conspiracy?

Since 1992, news reports have increasingly brought to the public's attention the possible health effects related to breast implants. Moreover, since the late 1980s, support and consumer advocacy groups have increasingly emerged, providing women who have received breast implants with more information about the potential dangers of these devices. Women who had made the decision to undergo surgery to enhance the size or shape of their breasts are now living with the uncertainty of not knowing how this decision will affect the rest of their lives. Two of the women I interviewed refer to themselves as "walking time bombs," as they fearfully anticipate the possibility of developing debilitating autoimmune problems. Others are already experiencing symptoms: aching joints, chronic fatigue, rashes, and hair loss—to name only a few.

The women I spoke with claimed that their plastic surgeons and the informed consent forms and information brochures handed to them prior to their surgeries led them to believe that the only possible dangers associated with implant mammaplasty were the risks of infection and anesthesia during the operation—risks common to any surgical procedure.[1] Less frequently, women said they were alerted to the possible occurrence of capsular contracture, the hardening of the implants caused by the formation of scar tissue. Apart from these warnings, plastic surgeons and the documents they provided either minimized or made no mention whatsoever of any other possible long-term health effects. Women also stated that they were not alerted to the possibility of implant rupture or leakage, which, in some cases, has led to multiple surgeries, scarring and disfigurement. Why were women not informed of all these risks?

In response to this question, most of the women I interviewed believed that their plastic surgeons neglected to inform them of the risks associated with breast implants because they were afraid that if they did, they would scare away potential patients and risk losing profits.[2] Women did not view their surgeons as the only culprits, but rather, they perceived them as being among the many players in a larger corporate and governmental conspiracy. They believed that individual doctors, along with implant manufacturers and government agents, all had "self-interest" in mind when they withheld knowledge about implant-related risk from the public.[3]

Women's explanations for why they were misinformed of the dangers associated with breast implants resonate with scholarly, political-economic critiques of the American health care system, which focus on the roles of power, control, greed, and profits to explain the troubles embedded within our current health care system. Many researchers, for instance, have explored the overlaps between corporate profits and industry-government connections.[4] Alexandra Dundas Todd provides a couple of examples:

> 1) In the 1980s the CEO for the parent company of Hooker Chemical Company (of Love Canal fame) was also the head of the President's Cancer Panel; and 2) the board of overseers for Sloan-Kettering Cancer Center, the largest private cancer center in the world, draws almost a third of its members from the chemical, oil, and car industries, and another third are leading financiers; other board members include drug company executives and, incredibly, tobacco industry barons.[5]

Some scholarship suggests that those who create these types of arrangements in the political economy continue to do so simply because they profit tremendously from them.[6] But, while profits and greed may explain part of the problem, Todd asserts that a political-economic critique of our health care system is "not enough. . . . The problem goes deeper than money." She states, "Belief systems also play a crucial role."[7]

Taking Todd's view in mind, a predominant belief in Western culture is that science and medicine are rational, objective, and value-neutral disciplines that perpetuate a reliance on a simplistic, linear, cause-and-effect model for treating the human body. Within this model, a plastic surgeon is perceived as a "healer," capable of improving a patient's self-esteem and self-confidence through medical procedures. But a plastic surgeon's expertise in molding, sculpting, and reshaping bodies also places him in the role of "artist." Together, these two roles are laden with assumptions about medicine, science, and gender.

A plastic surgeon possesses the ability to improve a woman's self-worth only in a cultural context in which women are defined in terms of their bodily attributes. In American society, where a woman's sense of femininity and selfhood is intrinsically linked to the size and shape of her breasts, plastic surgeons can perpetuate ideal female bodies while providing women with breast implants to "cure" their feelings of inadequacy. However, a plastic surgeon can "treat" a woman's poor sense of body image only because he is a trained, medical expert who works within a context that reflects the view that medical science is an objective and value-free discipline that holds the power to solve health-related problems through quick, simple, and safe medical interventions. Within this context, physicians are "trained to be healers, not harmers."[8] Taking these predominating beliefs into account, it becomes clearer why some plastic surgeons are so willing to dismiss or ignore problems related to implants, and thus fail to inform prospective implant candidates of possible dangers associated with the devices. For plastic surgeons, to reconceptualize breast implants as potentially harmful to women is probably not an easy task, since questioning the device's safety is equivalent to questioning their medical specialty and their profession.

Women's Political-Economic Critiques of Medicine

The majority of women I interviewed were angry that they had been misled by their plastic surgeons into believing that implants are "safe" when, in fact, the devices are linked to numerous complications and harmful side effects. However, they did not simply direct blame at their individual plastic surgeons who gave them incomplete and inaccurate information; rather, they found fault with the entire medical care system for causing their troubles. These women understood how their personal experiences with these doctors were linked to larger, cultural, political and economic contexts. For instance, some women's critiques of medicine were reminiscent of traditional feminist arguments that view a male-dominated medical conspiracy at work within our health care system. Lorraine, for example, pointed toward sexism as a rationale for explaining why plastic surgeons failed to warn women of the possible dangers of silicone: "Money is at the root of this whole implant ordeal. And, if plastic surgeons can make a few thousand dollars off of me . . . because some idea has been perpetrated by some male that this is the way women have to look—must look. And all these young guys swallow that stuff. It's all the boys' gang. The whole story is nothing but—all men do is cover up for themselves. They want what they want and they are going to get it one way or the other. And, the hell with the ramifications." Implicit in Lorraine's criticism is the view that women are the passive victims of male manipulation. According to her, men in our society hold the power to create, perpetuate, and profit from ideal images of female attractiveness, whereas women succumb to these images because they are powerless.

Some women's reports of their experiences with their plastic surgeons echo social science literature that suggests that physicians do not take female patients seriously, and treat them as if they are incapable of understanding complicated medical explanations.[9] For instance, prior to receiving breast implants, Nina had asked her plastic surgeon if implants could dislodge or "break." Her plastic surgeon trivialized her concern: "[The surgeon] started to relate my question to this story about one of his patients who was out on a dance floor at some formal ball or something. All of a sudden, the implants just fell out of her right there on the floor at the ballroom in front of all of these people. You know, and I was aghast! And then he stopped and looked at me and just started laughing, saying, 'Of course [implants] don't dislodge.'" Nina attempted to be a well-informed consumer, asking her surgeon an appropriate question related to the surgery she was considering. Even though implant rupture is a serious complication associated with breast augmentation, Nina's surgeon responded to her question without even acknowledging the possibility of this risk. Instead, he trivialized her concern with a fictitious account of a woman whose implants simply "fell out" of her body, and then he laughed at Nina's inquiry. In effect, he made Nina feel as though she had asked a foolish and inappropriate question.

While some of the women I interviewed understood their experiences with plastic surgeons in light of prevailing cultural assumptions about gender and power, others saw their medical encounters in a broader economic context. These women believed that power and greed were the culprits behind their receiving inaccurate and misleading information about implant safety. For instance, after experiencing joint pain and chronic fatigue, Sophie believed that her plastic surgeon failed to warn her of the risks associated with silicone because, "for plastic surgeons, providing women with implants is a big business. It is not to cure people. It is like these doctors are doing this intentionally to get people more sick so that they can get more business." According to Sophie, plastic surgeons and other physicians are more concerned about profiting from their patients' illnesses than they are about improving their patients' health and well-being.

Alice also claimed that her plastic surgeon neglected to inform her of any risks associated with breast implants. In order to make sense of why she was not provided with accurate information, she linked her personal experience to the political and economic structure of American society: "I just wonder if maybe the health industry somehow is connected with the tobacco industry [laughs], which is connected to the drug industry. The whole lot of them are in cahoots to keep the American public sick so that they can all make money—I don't know [laughs]. I wouldn't put it past them now." Alice explained that if she had known that her body would react to silicone, leading her to develop numerous health problems, she never would have gone through surgery to have implants. Finding fault with her physicians, she further stated, "But doctors, they just don't want to listen. They say, 'Oh, silicone is not reactive to the body.' Bullshit. Everything is reactive to the body at some point or another. And that's what makes me wonder. Are these [doctors] really men of science? They are not. They don't know what the hell they are talking about." Alice once trusted the medical profession to provide her with accurate information concerning health and illness, as well as about safety and risk associated with medical procedures and practices. Like many of the women I interviewed, she was disillusioned with the American medical system, which, according to her, is corrupted with capitalist, materialist ideals that evoke greed and power, even from her own doctors.

The medical and scientific literature is replete with information about the dangers associated with breast implants. For instance, reports indicate that implant-related complications may lead to multiple surgeries and possible disfigurement. Scientific studies have also called attention to potential long-term health problems associated with breast implants, such as connective-tissue diseases and autoimmune disorders. In light of this information about the risks associated with breast implants, it is no wonder that women blame their surgeons, implant manufacturers, and their government for misleading them down a path of supposed safety and security which, in reality, is fraught with medical uncertainty. Since breast implants were developed in the early 1960s, there have been questions about their safety and efficacy. It is this uncertainty around the risks associated with breast implants that has led me to a further examination of the interactive processes embedded in women's descriptions of their encounters with their plastic surgeons.

Alice told me that her surgeon failed to warn her of any potential problems associated with breast implants and accused the entire medical profession as being greedy and self-serving. Implicit in her accusation and her query ("Are not these [doctors] men of science?") are broader cultural assumptions shared by many of the women I talked with, about medicine, science, and physicians' roles within these disciplines. In Western society, medical science is presumed to be "pure," "accurate," and "certain"; therefore, "men of science" (or doctors) ought to possess "pure" "accurate," and "certain" knowledge about health and illness. Women visit their plastic surgeons because they are presumed to be "experts" of medical science who possess all the knowledge about risk and safety that is required to permit women to make informed choices about breast implantation. However, even "expert" knowledge about medical innovations or technologies is uncertain.[10]

A political-economic critique does not take into account cultural expectations of science and medicine. An examination of these expectations illuminates a deeper understanding of women's descriptions of their medical encounters and provides a more comprehensive explanation for why they were not informed of implant-associated risk. Furthermore, because breast size and shape have become so integral to a woman's self-concept as "feminine," it is also necessary to examine broader cultural ideas about women and the female body. The prevailing cultural and medical assumption is that providing women with more "normal"-looking bodies will improve their self-esteem and their self-confidence and will allow them to lead richer, fuller lives. Discussions between doctors and patients about the safety and risks associated with medical devices rarely occur without discussions of the benefits of these technologies. The benefits of receiving breast implants are intrinsically linked to a view of the ideal female body as perfectly proportioned and large-chested. Instances of physician neglect and manufacturer cover-ups clearly have perpetuated the misinformation that has been conveyed to women about the safety of breast implants. However, a conspiracy theory, or political-economic critique, ignores the dynamic interplay between cultural assumptions about gender and expectations for medical science. Consequently, these approaches fail to capture the complexity of how predominating views of medicine and science, and cultural ideas about femininity, womanhood, and the female body, infiltrate medical discourse, shaping the knowledge that is communicated to women by their physicians.

The work of social scientists has addressed this complex process. Emily Martin, for example, shows how current scientific thinking about the body as a complex system of interrelated, but "flexible," parts is used as a metaphor within larger organizational and institutional settings.[11] Martin began her research wondering "whether it would be possible to understand how the economic and social formation of late capitalism can influence 'culture,' in particular, internal and external forms of the body in health and illness."[12] But through the course of her investigation she discovered the impossibility of determining a causal link between "cultural" and "political economic" realms, and thus adopted in her analysis "a tactic of moving back and forth between descriptions of [these] realms."[13] Similarly, Susan Bell suggests that "metaphors from both the broad society and from within scientific and medical research communities move back and forth, reinforcing one another or creating tensions."[14] A political-economic critique of medicine assumes a causal relationship between greed and power, and misinformation about implant safety, yet ignores the complexity of the process through which tensions among the medical community, the implant industry, the government, and implant recipients are created and perpetuated. Ideas about femininity, womanhood, and female bodies, as well as assumptions about science and medicine, move back and forth among these groups, continually constructing and reconstructing knowledge about implant safety. This "knowledge," then, is disseminated to individual women by individual physicians within medical encounters. The FDA and the American Medical Association's negotiations around implant-related risk, and women's descriptions of their consultations with their plastic surgeons about the costs and benefits of implants shed light on this ongoing, interactive process. In the discussion that follows, I examine the implicit assumptions about femininity and female bodies that are embedded in the language of informed consent forms, information brochures, health care policy making, and women's descriptions of their medical consultations.

The Social Construction of "Costs and Benefits"

In 1978, when Rita was debating whether to undergo surgery to reconstruct her breast after a radical mastectomy, her plastic surgeon discussed with her the costs and benefits of receiving implants. During this consultation, he gave her a small brochure titled "Facts You Should Know about Your New Look," which reviews some commonly asked questions about breast implants. Rita had kept the brochure and showed it to me during my visit with her, explaining, "I used to keep everything that doctors give me." [15] The brochure clearly illustrates how assumptions about gender, medicine, and science transcend ideas about the risks and benefits associated with breast implants. The pamphlet, thus, provides an example of how "risks" and "benefits" are socially constructed. The brochure begins as follows: "If you are thinking about having breast implants, then join the hundreds of thousands of modern women who already have them. And hundreds of thousands more who will soon. Of course, you can look the way you wish. And be a totally happier woman. The procedure, when done by a qualified surgeon, is considered quite simple." [16] This passage conveys to women the message that receiving breast implants will not only improve their lives (by making them "happier"), but also will allow them participation in a larger social movement: Women can now "join the hundreds of thousands of 'modern' women" who are doing away with their old bodies in favor of breast enhancement. On an individual level, the passage conveys the message that cosmetic surgery can be perceived as a "liberating" experience, giving women more "choice" about how to present their outward appearances. On a broader cultural level, the reasoning embedded in the language of the brochure resonates with the perception of the body, as defined by Susan Bordo, as "cultural plastic" or, "a construction of life as plastic possibility and weightless choice undetermined by history, social location, or even biography." [17] According to Bordo, popular culture applies no brakes to fantasies of body alteration. In such a context, surgical breast enhancement not only is a simple route to happiness, but a woman can choose breasts that will look however she chooses—there are no limits implied by the brochure Rita showed me.

Like Bordo, I argue that a woman's decision to undergo surgery for body enhancement or alteration operates within a larger structural and cultural context that is shaped by assumptions about gender and medical science. In the passage presented in the brochure, a "modern," "happier" woman is one who has larger breasts, implying that a woman who does not partake in the massive trend toward body alteration is somehow "behind the times." The passage also conveys the message that there is a technical solution to a woman's problem of unhappiness—surgical breast enhancement. Only when performed by a "qualified surgeon" is this procedure simple, suggesting that only medical experts can provide women with the happiness achievable solely through plastic surgery.

In addition to answering questions about the surgical procedure itself, the pamphlet also addresses questions regarding the safety of implants. Despite evidence of implant leakage and rupture dating as far back as the early 1970s,[18] the 1976 brochure reads: "Based on laboratory findings and human experiences to date, a gel-filled breast implant should last for a lifetime."[19] Similarly, with regard to the risk of cancer it reads, "in the hundreds of thousands of cases where breast implants have been used, there have been no reported cases where cancer was attributed to the implant."[20] Finally, the pamphlet explains that since implants are placed between the pectoral muscle, they "do not interfere with the normal functioning of the milk ducts"—breast-feeding is therefore perfectly safe.[21] Although no long-term scientific studies had ever been conducted to determine how long implants last, or whether the devices pose a threat to women and their children's health, these statements indicate that the risk of implant-associated complications or damages is practically nil. Given what is known today about the frequency of implant rupture and other possible health problems related to silicone, it is striking that the statements in this information brochure are written in such a definitive tone. Yet, in Western society, medical knowledge is presumed to be clear-cut, black and white, absolute. These assumptions leave no room for questions about risk and safety. In fact, the only risk mentioned in Rita's information pamphlet was the possibility of infection during surgery. The document states nothing about the chance of rupture, nor the possibility of developing immunological or connective-tissue diseases. Perhaps mention of these "uncertain" dangers would not only scare away women who were entertaining the idea of breast alteration, but would also dissolve some of the predominating beliefs about medicine and science within our culture.

The information presented to Rita about the costs and benefits of breast implants during her initial visit with her plastic surgeon reflects larger cultural assumptions about femininity and womanhood, as well as prevailing ideas about science and medicine. As her pamphlet indicates, the perceived benefits of breast implants (improving women's self-esteem, self-confidence, and making women "happier") are intrinsically related to the ideal of the female body as large-breasted. Furthermore, the definitive tone of the pamphlet as it discusses the risks and safety associated with breast implants reflects larger cultural beliefs about medical and scientific knowledge as accurate and certain, despite the fact that knowledge about breast implants always has been vague and ambiguous.

Risks and Benefits, "Cosmetic" and "Reconstructive" Procedures

Like Rita, most of the women I interviewed claimed that their plastic surgeons provided them with misleading information about both the short- and long-term risks associated with breast implants prior to their surgeries. Some women said that they had held such high expectations of medicine, and placed so much faith in their plastic surgeons, that they never inquired about implant safety. Women who placed such trust in their plastic surgeons tended to be women who had had mastectomies.[22] For instance, Mary said that she trusted her doctors after she had her bilateral mastectomy, and felt no reason to question the safety of implants before her reconstructive surgery: "I didn't ever ask any questions like 'Now is this—do these [implants] wear out? Do they ever burst? Do they ever do anything like that?' I just figured the implants were permanent and that there were no problems because [my doctors] didn't tell me anything." Similarly, Brenda did not inquire about the risks associated with the implant she was to receive following her mastectomy. She explained, "It would be like going in to buy tires. To really know Michelin, Goodyear. Do you know all these brand names? Do

you know one hundred percent what they all do, what their perfor-
mance is? Why should I have to know all this information? Would you
not trust your plastic surgeon?" The language Brenda uses to describe
her trust in doctors reflects the dominant medical model. Within this
model, bodies are perceived as machines to be manipulated and managed
by medical experts. In light of this metaphor, Brenda's comment implies that just as mechanics are presumed to know everything about tires,
so, too, are plastic surgeons assumed to know everything about breast
implants.

In 1986, after Brenda learned that she had breast cancer, her oncologist sent her immediately to a plastic surgeon. Upon hearing that she
would have to undergo a mastectomy, Brenda explained that she was
"in a state of shock," incapable of comprehending her plastic surgeon's
description of the lengthy procedure involved with breast reconstruction. Only after she had a deflated silicone bag (or skin expander) implanted behind the skin of her concave chest wall, did she realize how
time-consuming and costly breast reconstruction can be for a mastectomy patient. The skin expander served as an elastic balloon between
her skin and chest wall, which was increasingly filled up with water
through an exterior valve.[23] For an entire year, Brenda had to make
regular weekly visits to her plastic surgeon's office to receive saline injections into her breast. Once Brenda's skin was sufficiently stretched
out, she had to undergo yet another operation for the removal of the
skin expander and the insertion of her silicone implant. Brenda's insurance company reimbursed her for her breast reconstruction but did
not compensate her for the travel expenses she accrued visiting her
plastic surgeon every week.[24] In Brenda's words, breast reconstruction
for a mastectomy patient is "time-consuming, it is expensive, and it is
painful."

Unlike Mary, who continued to trust her plastic surgeon, Brenda, in
hindsight, found fault with the medical profession for not adequately
informing her of the risks involved with implants, nor of the length and
time involved in the process of breast reconstruction. She explained,
"Would not it have been better [for the surgeon to have shown] me a
simplified film [on breast reconstruction]—something that I could understand in A, B, C layman language? Or, was it something that physicians enjoy—being in their private world, not really wanting to share
information with just a patient?" Yet, while Brenda pointed her finger

at the medical profession, she also explained how the nature of science and medicine within our culture played into her physicians' behavior, as well as her own feelings about the procedure she was undergoing:

> There is a zest, there is a zeal, the excitement of reconstructing my breast after a mastectomy conveyed to me by my doctors—that did make the difference in my decision [to have breast reconstruction]. And, I did have high regards for that medical, sterile world. I can recall being in the hallway of the clinic and my X ray was put up and men gathering around it, reading it—and the excitement of the cancer growing. [Breast cancer, and reconstruction] were things that these men were having symposiums on, they were sharing information, they were on the horizon of a medical extravaganza. I felt like a pioneer at one point in time. I felt as though I was physically and actively being a role model, and encouraged to be a role model for my daughter and the rest of women should this happen to. I was no longer just a patient. I was more than that. I was being psychologically conditioned do "do well" with [the reconstructive procedure], and to please. In fact, if you weren't doing well, you almost didn't want to say you weren't doing well.

Brenda explained that her own expectations of the "sterile" world of medicine and medical science combined with her physicians' own excitement about the discovery of her illness and the possibility of being able to reconstruct her breast, led her to become "psychologically dependent" on her physicians, and her reconstructive procedure. Feeling like a role model for other women experiencing breast cancer, she could not bear to disappoint her doctors by letting them know that she was actually experiencing a great deal of pain and discomfort. Confessing such problems to her doctors, and to herself, would be admitting that her own expectations of medicine as sterile, pure, and accurate were false, and that her faith in her physicians had been misguided.

One explanation for why mastectomy patients tended not to question their plastic surgeon's knowledge of implant-related risk may relate to these women's prior history with the medical profession. The women who had undergone reconstructive surgery after a mastectomy had reason to trust the medical profession: In most cases, it was their doctors who had detected their cancer and who restored them to good health— why should they discontinue respecting their physicians' opinions and advice concerning reconstructive surgery?

Another explanation for this finding may lie in the distinction between two separate rationales for procedures involving breast implants. For women who received implants following mastectomies, reconstructive surgery was perceived as more legitimate or "medically necessary," than surgery involving implants for "cosmetic" reasons. According to many of these women, undergoing a surgical procedure for the purpose of enlarging one's breasts is a matter of vanity; whereas having one's breast reconstructed after losing it to cancer is a matter of necessity— women facing the imminent loss of a part of their body that is intrinsically linked to their sense of femininity view themselves as having little choice but to restore their diseased bodies back to normalcy.[25] This perception may contribute to the less vigorous search for information about the risks associated with breast implants among those who had implants following mastectomies than among those who chose implants for cosmetic reasons.

Viewed by both surgeons and women as a procedure that allows breast cancer patients to move forward in their lives, breast reconstruction has become an integral part of the cancer recovery process. Indeed, most of the women I interviewed who had breast reconstruction following mastectomies continued to hold the medical profession in high regard, despite the lack of information given to them prior to their receiving implants. Kate, who had two implants after a bilateral mastectomy when she was sixty-four, stated: "I don't blame those doctors, because the ones that I had were very competent and they were trying to do a good job. They were faced with a difficult problem [her cancer]. And, the surgeon I had never does cosmetic surgery, he just does the surgery for cancer patients." Kate's comment illustrates how conceptualizing two separate rationales for procedures involving breast implants can lead to a perceived distinction between doctors who perform these procedures; surgeons who perform implant mammaplasty for "reconstructive" purposes are viewed as "legitimate," while those who perform the surgery for "cosmetic" reasons are seen as, in a sense, "illegitimate." With this reasoning, Kate came to believe that only those women who were under the substandard care of surgeons performing "cosmetic" surgeries experience problems with their implants: "Now, as I see it, people are more apt to have problems with their implants if they go to a plastic surgeon who does the surgery for appearance, not for *health* reasons." Even though many plastic surgeons perform both reconstructive and cosmetic surgeries involving breast implants, and women who receive implants for both reconstructive and cosmetic reasons experience implant-associated health problems and complications,

Kate finds comfort in conceptualizing a separation between her own experience with implants following breast cancer and the experiences of women who had implants for "other reasons."

Similarly, Maureen, who had a breast implant after the removal of her left breast when she was in her mid-fifties, believed that the women who say they are experiencing problems with implants are women who had implants for purely "cosmetic" reasons. "I think that maybe the candidates who are being given these implants maybe should be considered. I mean, I think that some of these women who are go-go dancers just look like they may have had all kinds of other diseases before they even decided to get breast augmentation. So, I think that it is kind of too bad to compare a woman like that to a woman who is your ordinary housewife, mother, what have you—who lives a more general, acceptable lifestyle, than someone who is. . . . There are so many variables that it is awfully hard to come to a conclusion." Embedded in this comment are elements of disapproval and blame. Maureen's words convey the view that women who receive implants for "reconstructive" purposes are good, virtuous, and moral; whereas women who have implants to enlarge their breasts are bad, impure, and oversexed. The good-girl/bad-girl dichotomy enables Maureen to castigate those women who have implants for breast enhancement as "bad," suggesting that their personal transgressions are to blame for their health problems. This type of lifestyle attack is also reflected in breast implant litigation and current research protocols. Although the scientific evidence concerning the risks associated with breast implants does not vary with regard to the type of procedure performed, plaintiffs who had reconstructive surgery with breast implants have been far more successful at winning individual lawsuits against implant manufacturers than women who had the surgery for cosmetic reasons. Like Maureen, juries may perceive reconstructive surgery as a legitimate, standardized medical procedure, separate from surgery performed on women who lead less "acceptable" lifestyles and go under the knife simply for the sake of appearances. Implicit in the logic that guides this distinction is the notion that the more "medical" the procedure appears, the less likely it will be perceived as "risky."

A recent study published in the *Journal of the American Medical Association* also attacks the lifestyles of women who have breast implants for augmentation purposes.[26] Linda Cook and her colleagues examined selected characteristics of 3,570 women, 80 of whom had breast implants for "cosmetic" reasons. The results of the research indicate that women with breast enlargements tend to drink more, have more sex partners, use oral contraceptives, and dye their hair more than the general female population. Not only do these findings imply that women with breast augmentations are "bad" girls, but they also may have severe implications for women who are sick and truly believe that their illnesses are caused by their implants. The authors of the study write: "Our results highlight the importance of careful consideration and evaluation of potential confounding variables when investigating the impact of breast augmentation on the risk of subsequent disease." [27] If future research protocols continue to focus on the lifestyles of women with implants, rather than on women's reports of the progression of symptoms they began to experience after receiving these devices, women may never find validation for their troubles.

Descriptions of "Risk" and "Safety" within Medical Encounters

Women's accounts of their interactions with their plastic surgeons suggest that their knowledge about implant-related risk is not necessarily related to the extent to which they actively elicit information from their doctors. For instance, since Jenna was so apprehensive about receiving breast implants, she asked her plastic surgeon numerous questions about implant safety prior to her surgery. Before her consultation with her plastic surgeon, she even conducted her own research on implant safety and found an article in a medical journal stating that silicone could cause cancer in rats. Concerned by this, she presented the article to her plastic surgeon, whose response was, "Well, rats get tumors from anything." Jenna also asked her surgeon about the durability of implants. Her surgeon attempted to reassure her by trivializing her concern, "If you were in a car accident, the implants would probably save your life."

Similarly, Eve asked her plastic surgeon a number of questions related to implant safety. She recalled:

> I asked [my plastic surgeon] how long the implants would last, and he told me that when I died, fifty years after I died, when they opened my coffin, my breast implants would look exactly the way they did when he put them in. And I had asked him about the risks such as punctures—what would happen if I got in a car accident? I asked him some pretty intelligent questions—the

possibility of leakage. He said, "Actually, the only way that these are ever going to leak is if someone actually stabbed you with a knife." I asked him about the possibility of being able to nurse. He said, "No problem." Loss of sensation—"No problem."

Beth, who received her implants in 1981, also explained that she tried to gather as much information as possible on breast implants before she went ahead with the procedure: "I did as much research as I could— you know, being what I thought was responsible. I interviewed several different surgeons and asked them if there were any problems connected with the implants. I asked, 'Are there any complications involved in doing this? Any risks whatsoever?'" However, she said, "The only thing that these surgeons told me was that the implants sometimes encapsulate and that all you would have to do in this case is have a surgeon squeeze hard and bust the capsule. I had a surgeon do this many times." In her statement, Beth was referring to the procedure called a "closed capsulotomy," a procedure that has been found to rupture implants and is no longer recommended by the FDA or the American Society of Plastic and Reconstructive Surgeons as a standardized form of care. And yet, in Beth's description of her interaction with her plastic surgeon, a closed capsulotomy is intended to alleviate or minimize implant-related problems, not compound them. Moreover, the procedure was presented to Beth as a completely logical and straightforward medical practice. However, her own experience suggests that the procedure was quite painful. The language Beth used to describe it ("squeezing hard" to "bust" the capsule) indicates that, from the layperson's perspective, a closed capsulotomy may even be considered harmful. The voice of medicine, however, strips away this context of meaning.

The history of information about the risks associated with closed capsulotomies illustrates again the fact that elements of uncertainty are commonly found in medicine and that knowledge about medical procedures and treatments is always evolving. This point is also reflected in the information that has been shared about the risks associated with various kinds of breast implants. Carmen was considering breast implants in 1992. Because she had listened to news reports about the risks associated with the silicone prosthesis, she wanted to know if similar dangers pertained to the saline implant. She explained, "I asked [my plastic surgeon], 'Are the risks with the saline similar to the silicone?'" Her surgeon responded, "No. It is just water and salt—what harm could that do your body?" During this interaction, no mention was made of the fact that even saline implants are surrounded by a silicone envelope, which may lead to health problems similar to those caused by the silicone device, nor was there mention of the possibility of implant deflation—a common occurrence among saline implants. To this day, Carmen is still unaware of any risks associated with her saline breast implants.[28]

In 1990, when Alice visited her plastic surgeon to ask questions about the different types of breast implants available to women, he gave her a very different impression of the risks and benefits associated with each prosthesis than was conveyed to Carmen by her doctor. Alice recalled that her surgeon advised her against the saline prosthesis, telling her, "'Saline doesn't last that long. After five years, seven years, you are going to have to come back and I'm going to have to put new ones in. You don't want to have all these operations do you?' And I said, 'No.' And he goes, 'Well, silicone will last until you are old and gray and you will have the perkiest breasts ever, they won't disintegrate.'"

Carmen and Alice's plastic surgeons had diverging views about which types of implants involved the least amount of risk and were the most effective. In Alice's case, her surgeon's knowledge about the frequency of rupture with the saline implants, compounded with his perception of the advantage of silicone implants (they could give Alice the "perkiest breasts ever"), led to his convincing Alice that she would be "better off" if she received the silicone devices. Carmen received her implants in 1992 during the height of the public controversy over silicone implants. Aware that these implants were potentially harmful, Carmen opted for saline implants after her plastic surgeon reassured her that these implants could do no harm since they were "just water and salt." The conflicting information plastic surgeons convey to their patients about the costs and benefits associated with various types of implants reveals the extent to which knowledge about risk involving medical technologies is uncertain, ambiguous, and continuously evolving.

Interactions between the FDA, the Medical Community, and Implant Manufacturers

Many women I interviewed were not only angry with their plastic surgeons for leading them to believe that they were receiving a perfectly harmless medical device, but some also found fault in the FDA for taking a hands-off attitude toward the regulation of breast implants. In fact, all of the women I interviewed explained that prior to their surgeries, they were not even aware that breast implants had never been approved for medical use by the FDA.[29]

In the late 1980s and early 1990s, evidence of long-term risks associated with implants increasingly surfaced in medical and scientific journals. Prior to the media coverage of these studies women and many plastic surgeons were unaware of potential problems associated with these devices. A staff report on the FDA's regulation of breast implants suggests that manufacturer fraudulence and plastic surgeons' negligence were the chief reasons why information about the dangers of implants was never disseminated to the public. For instance, the congressional committee investigating this report found that in the 1970s, Dow Corning misled plastic surgeons to believe that it had conducted all the necessary testing to conclude that implants are safe, when in fact these claims were based only on a two-year dog study.[30] The committee also discovered that Medical Engineering Corporation, the breast implant manufacturer, which was later bought out by Bristol-Myers Squibb, withheld results of a beagle study that indicated adverse reactions to silicone, including "hemorrhage, possible pneumonia of the lung, and hyperplasia of lymphoid tissue in the large intestines."[31] In response to these results, the president of the company demanded that the dogs be sacrificed and their organs be disposed of immediately.[32]

According to the committee's report, plastic surgeons were also at fault for never demanding proof of implant safety from manufacturers. Instead, surgeons erroneously placed their faith in the information conveyed to them by representatives from these companies. They distributed information brochures to their patients that say little, if anything, about the short- or long-term complications and health risks linked to implants.

In 1988, an FDA advisory panel met and decided that patients receiving breast implants were not being adequately warned of the risks involved with these devices. To rectify the situation, the FDA convened a group of representatives from among plastic surgeons, implant manufacturers, and consumer groups to develop a voluntary information brochure that would list all the risks associated with implants. When the devices were pulled from the market in 1992, the brochure still had not been approved,[33] indicating that a consensus could not be reached as to what constituted implant-related "risk" and what did not.

A predominating belief in our culture is that the methods employed by medicine and modern science are capable of measuring and determining the truth. However, this belief is met with opposing views from social scientists who contend that even scientific knowledge is socially constructed[34] and that scientific outcomes are continuously negotiated.[35] The inability of the FDA, plastic surgeons, implant manufacturers, and consumer groups to develop an information brochure on the risks associated with breast implants reflects conflicts within this negotiation process. According to the committee's staff report on the government regulation of implants, the FDA was fully aware of the potential problems related to silicone leakage, rupture, and migration. Plastic surgeons and implant manufacturers, however, had a vested interest in keeping the device on the market. Both of these groups were profiting tremendously from the production and distribution of the devices. Plastic surgeons also believed that the device indeed was benefiting women, since so many women continued to come to their offices asking for implants in order to feel better about their bodies and to improve "self-esteem" or "self-confidence." Surgeons were doing a service for women and in the end were convinced that the FDA should take a back-seat role on the issue of implant safety.

The committee's staff report further claims that even after concerns about the potential dangers of silicone were revealed by Dow Company memoranda in February 1992, and by further scientific studies conducted in recent years, the American Society of Plastic and Reconstructive Surgeons (ASPRS) and the American Medical Association (AMA) continued to minimize implant-related risks to their patients. These risks were downplayed in informed consent forms presented to women.[36]

In the late 1980s and early 1990s, the FDA drafted an informed consent form for plastic surgeons to use to explain the procedure to their patients prior to their surgery. This document listed all the possible complications and health effects associated with breast implants, including frequency of ruptures, silicone leakage, connective-tissue disease, autoimmune problems, and interference with mammography and breast-feeding. However, representatives from the ASPRS and the AMA complained that this form would raise unnecessary concerns among women and that it went beyond the known risks, referring to studies that had yet to be conducted.[37]

The AMA and ASPRS's dissatisfaction with the original informed consent form prompted the FDA to revise the original version of the document, minimizing the risks associated with the device. For instance, the FDA weakened warnings associated with breast-feeding. The original informed consent form read: "The surgical implantation of the device may interfere with a woman's ability to nurse her baby. . . . Although this is a known risk, the extent of the risk is not known."[38] The revised document states: "Many women with breast implants have nursed their babies successfully. . . . Any breast surgery, including breast implant surgery, could theoretically interfere with your ability to nurse your baby."[39] Similarly, the original document stated that implants may rupture and that "silicone gel may migrate to the surrounding breast tissue and other parts of the body." The revised version states: "The gel released as a result of rupture may be contained within the capsule surrounding the implants. If the scar envelope also tears, the gel can travel (migrate) and be squeezed into the breast tissue or into the muscle or fatty tissue next to the breast, abdominal wall, or arm. Fortunately, this is uncommon. The risks from this escaped gel are unknown."[40] According to the staff report, this statement is misleading: Implant rupture rates range from 0 to 32 percent; implants over ten years old are almost always ruptured when removed from a patient; and studies have never been conducted on gel migration through a torn capsule—therefore, the statement that this is "uncommon" is unfounded.[41]

Only four of the forty women I interviewed received implants either in 1990 or thereafter. Six of the women I interviewed had their implants replaced after 1990. All ten of these women reported that they were shown informed consent forms prior to receiving implants. Tracy recalled that the form contained a list of all the risks associated with implants, including the possibility of implant rupture and leakage, as well as the possible autoimmune problems that may result from silicone. However, Tracy also claimed that the wording in the document made these risks seem highly uncommon. Moreover, her plastic surgeon minimized any potential dangers related to the device. With regard to risk related to mammography, Tracy explained, "Basically, the booklet said that there is more difficulty reading a mammogram. But they can compensate for it by giving you extra views. Instead of giving you the four normal views of a breast, you would get like six. You still didn't see all the tissue, but they lead you to believe in the conversation and in the pamphlet that you saw most of it—whatever that means." By 1992, after the risks related to implants had been widely publicized, Tracy decided to conduct her own investigation of implant-related risk.

Through her research, she discovered that breast implants can obscure up to 80 percent of all breast tissue during mammography, and explained, "Eighty percent would have been enough to get me off the chair and walking . . . because I have always been concerned about my health." In fact, all of the women I interviewed who were aware of the risks associated with implants (all but Carmen) explained that if they had been fully informed of these risks, they would never have traded their health for their appearance.[42]

Tracy further recalled reading the form mentioning risks related to implant rupture and autoimmune disease, but explained that "the [plastic surgeon] told me that he had put in several hundred implants every year and he has only had one that ruptured. So, it sounded like these things never—hardly ever, ever rupture. And as far as getting lupus or getting autoimmune diseases, he has never had a person come down with that—and, 'there is no association with silicone and autoimmune diseases.' . . . And, it sounded like—except for the fact that having surgery—it sounded like a relatively risk-free operation in terms of getting this desired result, you know, improving my image and so forth."

Conveying his own beliefs about the costs and benefits of implants, Tracy's plastic surgeon relied on his own experience as a physician (the fact that he "only had one [case of] rupture," and "never had a person come down with [autoimmune disease after receiving an implant]") as evidence that breast implants are safe. This information confirmed his belief that implant safety is known and certain and validated his role as artist and physician: He could give Tracy her "desired result" and improve her self-image by altering her breast size.

A medical conspiracy theory posits that the AMA and ASPRS's dissatisfaction with the original informed consent form and plastic surgeons' reluctance to disclose accurate information about implant safety to their patients are linked to a larger political and economic context, suggesting that the medical community intentionally withheld information regarding implant safety because physicians were afraid of losing profits. However, missing from this explanation is a consideration of how cultural assumptions about gender and medical science transcend these tensions between the medical community and the FDA.

The AMA and ASPRS's recommendations for changes on the original version of the informed consent form reflect physicians' own unwillingness to perceive science and medicine as uncertain, uncontrolled, or vague endeavors. In the case of risk associated with breast-feeding, the words "the extent of risk is unknown" in the original document, were changed to words reflecting more certainty: "many women have nursed their babies successfully." In other cases, words pointing toward uncertainty are used only when an event is "rare." For instance, in the case of a rupture "the risks from escaped gel are unknown," but "fortunately [the chance of gel escaping] is uncommon."[43] This statement reinforces the idea that medical science and plastic surgeons work together to create female bodily perfection and help women feel better about themselves, improving their "self-esteem."

As both "physicians" and "artists," plastic surgeons operate within a context that is laden with assumptions about medicine, science, and gender. Over the past thirty years, within American society, plastic surgery has given way to an entirely new perspective on outward appearances. This perspective assumes an ideal body type for men and women and justifies its practices on the premise that outward appearance affects quality of life. Assumptions about gender pervade this logic. For instance, the prevailing assumption about women and breast size is that women who have larger, more shapely breasts are perceived as more sexual, or more "feminine"; therefore, surgical procedures to enhance women's breasts are expected to improve women's self-concept as female.

Assumptions about medical science also pervade this logic. In her discussion on perspectives of childbirth, Barbara Katz Rothman claims that the predominant obstetrical (or medical) perspective continues to be held as "the truth. . . . We believe our medicine has the *facts*."[44] Similarly, as surgery to change outward bodily appearances becomes more popular, individuals are increasingly relying on plastic surgeons for the "facts" about beauty and attractiveness. As artists and as scientists and healers practicing within the medical model, plastic surgeons are expected by women to hold all the answers about what constitutes a beautiful body. Similarly, women wishing to alter the size or shape of their breasts assume plastic surgeons know what is best for them. As trained medical experts, plastic surgeons themselves may believe they have all the answers about health, illness, and what constitutes desirable gendered traits. These assumptions leave little room for uncertainty and risk about the medical devices that plastic surgeons use to mold and reshape individual bodies or, perhaps more important, to improve the quality of their patients' lives. For plastic surgeons, these perceived benefits may far outweigh any uncertain risks related to breast implants:

To question the safety of the tools of their trade is to question their medical and professional roles as scientists, artists, and healers.

There is a sense of certainty and simplicity to the logic. If a woman feels self-conscious about her body, a plastic surgeon can improve her self-image by providing her with a new one. With their years of medical training, plastic surgeons have earned their title as "healers." To women feeling badly about their breast size or shape, these doctors appear to possess the skill, expertise, and tools needed to make women's emotional pain and discomfort around poor body image disappear. Moreover, after women view the remarkable difference between the before-and-after photos presented to them in their plastic surgeons' offices[45] and are told that breast implants are safe, they become even further caught up in the idea that body alteration and enhancement with implants will improve their lives. Rose explained, "The doctors made it seem like implants were the greatest thing since ice cream." Similarly, Grace stated that since her plastic surgeon told her that implants were safe and the procedure simple, "breast implants were like a carrot being dangled in front of me." For these women, as well as their plastic surgeons, breast implants were perceived as a quick, simple and seemingly safe solution to improving self-esteem and self-confidence.

However, often left unquestioned is a missing piece to the reasoning that plastic surgeons can serve as both "healers" and "artists." Considering again the before-and-after comparisons presented to women in their plastic surgeons' offices prior to their surgeries, this missing link becomes ever so obvious. In the photos, the heads of the women are absent, and so too are their identities. Plastic surgeons are not healing *women*, nor the source of their problems; rather, they are treating fragmented body parts—only women's breasts appear in the photos.

As many women came to realize that the risks associated with breast implants may be far greater than what was told to them by their plastic surgeons, they began to call into question not only the information that was conveyed to them by their plastic surgeons, but also the role of the plastic surgeon (or the informer) himself. After Karen realized that her deteriorating health could be related to her implants, she came to view plastic surgeons not as healers but solely as "artists" whose presumed role is to enable women adhere to ideal beauty standards: "I don't think that [implanting women with a potentially dangerous medical device] was a malicious or calculated effort on the part of plastic surgeons. It was more 'Well, women want bigger breasts, and this is my role.' A lot of plastic surgeons see themselves as these artists, and we, as women, become an extension of them—a trophy for them." The perception of plastic surgeons as artists enabled Karen to understand these doctors' practices within a larger cultural context. Within this context, the female body is just a piece of art or a "trophy" for those who possess the ability to sculpt and mold her. Christine also came to perceive an incongruity between the role of plastic surgeon as "healer" and the role of plastic surgeon as "artist." As she reflected back on the lack of information she was provided about implant-related risk, she remarked, "I don't think that plastic surgeons are doctors or healers, I think they are exterior decorators."

6

Minimizing Women's Troubles

*T*hirty-four of the forty women who participated in this study explained that after receiving breast implants, they began experiencing a variety of symptoms ranging from sleep disturbances and stomach irritability to chronic fatigue and debilitating rheumatic disorders. Most of these women did not associate these symptoms with their breast implants until the early 1990s, after they began reading news reports or listening to television talk shows that focused on a potential relationship between implants and autoimmune disease. Frightened about their future health, these women turned to medicine hoping to disentangle the "medical facts" from "sensationalist media hype." Hillary, one of my respondents who used to work for a plastic surgeon, explained that after a segment about the dangers of breast implants aired on *Face to Face with Connie Chung*,[1] her office received over twenty-five calls a day for over a month from "frantic" implant recipients. Similarly, the women I interviewed said that when they first learned about the possible dangers associated with silicone, they were so alarmed that they immediately called their plastic surgeons or made appointments with rheumatologists, immunologists, and other specialists hoping to find out the "truth" about implant-related risk. These women had faith in medicine and trusted their physicians to provide them with accurate and definitive answers about health, illness, and disease causation. Nevertheless, they explained that the more they approached medical "experts" with questions about breast implants and their worsening symptoms, the more disillusioned and disappointed they became—rather than providing them with "reasonable" explanations to account for their deteriorating health, the physicians minimized and dismissed the women's fears and anxieties, as well as their physical symptoms.

Twenty-eight percent of the thirty-five women I interviewed who had experienced unexpected problems with their implants, such as ruptures and encapsulation, claimed that their physicians treated these complications as if they were normal, common side effects of breast implants that warranted no concern. Although some women initially felt reassured by this response, after they listened to news reports on the long-term health effects associated with migrating silicone from faulty implants, they became frightened and concerned. Many of these women eventually realized that what their physicians were labeling as "minor" problems were, in fact, signs of potentially serious trouble. For instance, plastic surgeons dealt with implant ruptures by telling women not to worry since the problem could easily be "fixed" by replacing their failed devices with "newer and improved" implants. Women, however, eventually learned that their ruptures may have put them at greater risk for developing autoimmune diseases and rheumatic disorders. Indeed, many of the women I interviewed whose implants had ruptured were already experiencing aching joints, hair loss, rashes, chronic fatigue, and other symptoms. Similarly, plastic surgeons responded to women's encapsulated implants by telling them that they should not be concerned since the problem could be resolved with a "quick" and "simple" medical procedure—a "closed capsulotomy." Women who had this procedure later discovered that it may have ruptured their implants.

Women also claimed that their physicians minimized their implant-related troubles by relegating them to the realm of psychological or emotional complaints. In fact, 23 percent of the thirty-four women in my sample who reported experiencing implant-related symptoms reported that they were referred to psychiatric care for treatment of these problems. Many of these women said that their doctors had diligently performed tests for lupus, Sjögren's syndrome, and various other immunological disorders; however, since the results of these lab reports almost always came back "normal," physicians were unable to attribute women's symptoms to any known medical or physiological condition.

Consequently, they proceeded to tell their patients that their real problems were in their heads, not in their bodies.

Finally, 22 percent of the thirty-four women I spoke with who believed they were experiencing implant-related illnesses reported that their physicians commonly misdiagnosed their symptoms with signs of less serious physical conditions. For instance, after experiencing intense pain in her chest, Rose went to the emergency room and was told that she had a mild case of costochondritis (inflammation of tissue surrounding the ribs) when, in fact, her body was rejecting her implant, which was trying to break through her chest wall. Similarly, Jenna had a rash across her stomach for two months and was told by her primary care physician that she had poison ivy. She now suspects that the rash was an indication of an allergic reaction to her implants. More commonly, women reported that their doctors confused their "silicone-related" symptoms with signs of menopause, premenstrual syndrome, or other "female" conditions and disorders.

In Chapter 5, I reported that many of the women I spoke with blamed their physicians for not informing them of the risks associated with breast implants. These women had a similar reaction toward their physicians after they began to realize that these practitioners were undermining and invalidating their implant-related health problems and concerns. These women were angry and disillusioned with medicine. They believed that their doctors were not only intentionally withholding information about implant-related risk but, in so doing, were also deliberately trivializing or ignoring their health problems for fear of lawsuits. Barbara stated, "I cannot remember any good experience or kindness from the medical profession in dealing with [my problems with implants]. I think they were sort of covering their mistakes and trying to cover their colleagues." Frances similarly commented, "[Doctors] don't want to talk about [breast implants]. They are afraid I think. They are afraid you are going to sue them if they give you something that makes you sick."

In Chapter 5, I argued that while finding fault with medical "culprits" may provide an outlet for women's anger, a "medical conspiracy" fails to take into account how larger cultural and institutional forces shape ideas about the risks and benefits associated with breast implants. Cultural assumptions about gender and societal expectations of science and medicine influence one another, continually reconstructing the knowledge about implant-related risk that is conveyed to women by their physicians. A conspiracy theory also ignores how the structure and organization of modern medicine in Western culture shapes physicians' responses to women's implant-related health problems and concerns. Just as assumptions about gender and expectations of medical science pervade ideas about implant risk, so, too, do they pervade beliefs about, and medical treatments for, women's implant-related symptoms and complications. Thus, while analyzing women's descriptions of their medical encounters, I argue that physicians' responses to their troubles with implants are not necessarily linked to a secret plan to keep women in the dark, but are actually typical of medicine stemming from three factors:

1. A reliance on the biomedical model that perceives illness as a distinctly biological phenomenon that can be scientifically measured and categorized
2. A trend toward increased specialization and technological determinism in medicine, which perpetuates the idea that disease causation can be explained by perceiving the human body as a conglomeration of fragmented and isolated parts to be mechanically manipulated and cured
3. A male bias in the production of scientific and medical knowledge, which has led to the assumptions that female bodies are inherently diseased and that women patients are innately overemotional

Minimizing Women's Problems: "It's No Big Deal"

Most of the women I interviewed reported experiencing unexpected complications with their breast implants. For instance, Jenna explained that about a month after she had received saline implants in 1989, her left implant dislodged and shifted up into her armpit. Other women informed me that immediately after their surgeries, their breasts became infected and inflamed. More commonly, my respondents reported that their implants eventually ruptured or encapsulated with scar tissue.

Women whose implants had ruptured had different theories to explain how this complication had occurred. For instance, several of the women I spoke with who had experienced capsular contracture had agreed to undergo a procedure known as a closed capsulotomy, which involves the forceful squeezing and twisting of the breast to break the hard fibrous scar tissue surrounding the implant. Some of these women believed that a closed capsulotomy had caused their ruptures.[2] Other women I interviewed believed that a mammogram or a blow to the chest had broken the envelope surrounding their implants. Finally, some of my respondents suspected that their implants had failed because the devices were so old that their exterior silicone envelopes had simply disintegrated.

Medical literature since the 1980s, as well as news reports over the past several years, has suggested that migrating silicone from ruptured or leaking breast implants can cause debilitating autoimmune diseases and rheumatic disorders. Moreover, a failed prosthesis may lead to the need for several operations, which can leave a woman severely scarred and disfigured: If a woman's implant has ruptured, she must have it removed; and if silicone has seeped into surrounding breast tissue, she may need to undergo another surgery to clean out the silicone. Some women also develop silicone granulomas in their breasts after their implants have either ruptured or leaked, requiring even further surgery.

The women I interviewed explained that when they had made the decision to have breast implants, they were not informed that these devices could break or leak silicone into their bodies. In fact, most of them reported that their plastic surgeons had led them to believe that breast implants were so durable that they would "last a life time." Consequently, when women learned that one or both of their implants had ruptured, they were alarmed and frightened. Women whose implants had unexpectedly hardened as a result of capsular contracture also were concerned and disappointed. Thinking that having implants would improve their appearances, these women ended up with breasts that resembled "tether balls" and "basketballs," or were "as hard as rock."

Despite the fear and anxiety women endured after experiencing these and other types of unforeseen complications, women reported that their physicians responded to their problems by treating them as normal and common side effects of breast implants which they expected women to tolerate. For instance, when Barbara's breasts had hardened after her surgery, she returned to her plastic surgeon, who told her, "That is the way your breasts are supposed to look."

Similarly, women explained that their doctors described the procedures and surgeries that were necessary to "fix" their implant-related problems as normal, safe, and standardized forms of care, when, in fact, they eventually led to further complications. For instance, while Jenna was startled when her implant had migrated from her chest to underneath her arm, she explained that her plastic surgeon was "very unimpressed" by her problem and treated it as if it were "no big deal." He simply told Jenna that he would replace her implants with silicone devices that were "less likely to move around and encapsulate." Trusting her surgeon's advice, Jenna agreed to this surgery. However, soon thereafter, she began to experience a wide range of strange symptoms, including chronic fatigue, fevers, and hair loss. Jenna now believes that these symptoms were associated with her body's immunological response to her "new and improved" implants.

Sheila reported that her surgeon also reacted as if the complication she had experienced with her implants was a normal occurrence. In 1973, about two months after she had undergone her cosmetic surgery, her breasts became extremely hard, painful, and uncomfortable. When she phoned her plastic surgeon about this problem, he told her that he could easily "fix" it by performing a closed capsulotomy. Just as Jenna trusted her surgeon's expertise, so, too did Sheila. Thinking that a closed capsulotomy was a safe and simple medical procedure, she went along with her surgeon's recommendation and allowed him to manually tug and pull at her breasts in order to "pop" the scar capsules surrounding her implants. Sheila said that the procedure was unexpectedly painful; nevertheless, she felt reassured by her visit: "The surgeon made it sound as if the hardening was minor—just something that happened from the surgery that was no big deal, and that this procedure [the closed capsulotomy] was just a standard procedure." In the early 1990s, after listening to media reports of the possible dangers of implants and after conducting her own research on implant-related risk, Sheila learned that a closed capsulotomy can rupture breast implants and, subsequently, lead to debilitating autoimmune diseases. About a year before I interviewed her, Sheila had an ultrasound of her breasts that indicated that her left implant was, in fact, ruptured. She suspected that the closed capsulotomy she had about twenty years earlier had caused this problem.

Another case is Grace, who, in 1971, had received one implant in her right breast to correct for a congenital deformity. About a year following, she noticed a small blister on her right breast and suspected that something was wrong with her implant. However, when she visited her plastic surgeon with this problem, he told her "not to worry," that her implant was "fine." Moreover, he explained that even if there was a problem with the device, it would be "no problem," because he could just "pop another one in." Grace accepted her doctor's assessment of her problem and went home feeling reassured. However, over the course of several years, she began noticing that her blister had grown significantly wider and deeper, while her breast had become smaller. In the early 1990s, Grace had learned that implants can slowly leak silicone into the body and can potentially cause autoimmune disorders and connective tissue diseases. After reading about these problems in the newspaper, she decided to call a local women's health collective, which provided her with a detailed list of all the reported symptoms experienced by implant recipients. Almost every symptom listed corresponded with her own long history of health troubles.

Many of the women I interviewed explained that they were angry with their physicians after learning that their ruptured and leaking implants had potentially put them at greater risk for developing disabling autoimmune diseases. How could these medical "experts" lead them to believe that the complications they were experiencing were "normal" and "common" side effects of breast implants when, in fact, they were signs of potentially serious trouble? In their efforts to answer this question, the women I spoke with directed blame at the medical community. They suspected that their physicians had known all along about the dangers associated with silicone and intentionally withheld information from them in order to protect their professional reputations. Christine, for example, explained, "I do not understand how so many bright doctors could look at this [breast implant] issue and not know that there is a problem. And, so they do know, they have to know. They are only defending their position to protect the political bias of the medical profession. . . . And, they have to maintain that the ways they treat problems with implants are routine, standards of care. Otherwise, a lot of doctors could get their asses sued. That is the bottom line really. So, they probably get together and laugh about it."

Some women described specific cases in which their doctors deliberately lied to them to cover up their mistakes. For example, Joyce explained that her plastic surgeon led her to believe that her implants were "fine" when, in fact, a mammogram and ultrasound she had undergone in 1991 both indicated an "unmistakable deformity" in one of her implants. She was unaware of these test results until she switched plastic surgeons in 1993. Her new doctor obtained her medical records and, after examining the two X rays of Joyce's breasts, immediately noticed the deformity. Subsequently, Joyce had a magnetic resonance image

(MRI) taken of her breasts, which confirmed that both of her implants were ruptured. In hindsight, she believes that her first plastic surgeon intentionally withheld important information from her in order to protect himself from a potential lawsuit.

Jane also believes that her plastic surgeon had deceived her. She explained that after her first set of silicone breast implants had ruptured, her surgeon told her that he would replace them with "safer" saline ones. Months after Jane's replacement surgery, her breasts became painful and lumpy. At around the same time, in December 1990, *Face to Face with Connie Chung* aired a segment about the dangers associated with silicone implants. Immediately after the show, Jane decided to call her plastic surgeon's office to reassure herself that the implants inside her body were not linked to any of the health effects reported in the media. However, instead of feeling relieved by her phone call, she was stunned—her surgeon's secretary informed her that she did not have saline implants, but polyurethane-covered, silicone-gel-filled devices. According to media reports, these implants were carcinogenic.[3] Jane later found out that the same surgeon who had lied to her about the type of implants he had given her also neglected to inform her that in the process of removing her ruptured implants, he had scraped out a large quantity of her breast tissue, which was contaminated with silicone. She explained, "He gave me a mastectomy and didn't even tell me." Not until Jane had her polyurethane-covered implants removed by a different surgeon was she informed that she had practically no tissue left in her breasts.

Frances similarly discovered years after she had her first set of implants removed that the physician who had performed this surgery had withheld important medical information from her. Frances had received silicone implants in 1977 following a bilateral mastectomy. By 1979, her implants had encapsulated, causing her breasts to become hard, painful, and deformed. To solve this problem, Frances's surgeon convinced her to have her silicone implants replaced with saline implants intended to prevent the recurrence of capsular contracture. In the early 1990s, Frances learned through reading her medical records that her silicone implants were ruptured. Her surgeon had never conveyed this information to her. Nevertheless, Frances was not angry. She simply explained, "Well, you know, back then, [ruptured implants] were probably no big deal."

Frances's comment implicitly points to the fact that, in the 1970s, leading medical journals had yet to address the safety of breast implants—the link between autoimmune disease and these devices was not widely publicized until the early 1990s. Prior to this time, only a small number of rheumatology and immunology journals had published research demonstrating a connection between silicone and rheumatic or immunological disorders.[4] Concerned with only the latest developments in their own field of specialization, most plastic surgeons probably were unaware of these studies,[5] and simply chose the type of implant they thought worked best. For many surgeons, this meant implanting women with devices that produced a good "cosmetic result" without rupturing or encapsulating. For instance, some surgeons used polyurethane-covered implants since their textured envelopes (which scientists later suspected to be carcinogenic) were assumed to prevent capsular contracture and produce a more natural feel than other implants on the market. However, by the 1990s, as scientific studies increasingly called into question the safety of these and other silicone-gel-filled implants, saline implants became the preferred implant among many plastic surgeons. Now, even these devices have come under scrutiny—the FDA has launched an investigation of their safety, and consumer advocacy groups are urging the government to restrict their use.

While some women's descriptions of their experiences with physicians point toward cases of medical malpractice, they also show how the knowledge about the risks and benefits associated with different types of implants has been continuously evolving. For instance, in the 1970s, Frances's surgeon had replaced her encapsulated silicone implants with saline ones that, according to him, were the "greatest" implants on the market. However, in the 1980s, Jenna's plastic surgeon dealt with her failed saline devices by replacing them with "better" silicone prostheses, which were less likely to shift around and become hard. And, in Jane's case, her surgeon in 1990 told her he was implanting her with new and improved "textured" implants (which, to her surprise, turned out to be silicone gel implants surrounded by a polyurethane, textured envelope).

Women's descriptions of their encounters with plastic surgeons illustrate how physicians deal with the ambiguous and uncertain qualities of medicine by dismissing as normal their patients' troubles. Rather than convey to women that the risks associated with breast implants are indefinite and vague, plastic surgeons responded to women's implant-related complications by telling them that the troubles they were experiencing were "no big deal," or were normal, common side effects that warranted no concern. Surgeons led women to believe that the procedures and surgeries used to treat encapsulated or ruptured implants were standardized and safe forms of care. However, women's accounts of their implant-related experiences indicate that the perceived risks and benefits of these medical interventions are uncertain.

Women's descriptions of their surgeons' responses to their implant-related problems suggest that medical knowledge is never definitive and complete. Nevertheless, the dominant medical perspective in Western society perpetuates the belief that physicians are supposed to know everything they need to know about the devices they use and the procedures they perform. Working within this belief system, physicians may not intentionally withhold information from their patients, but may unwittingly conceal their lack of knowledge about the seriousness of their patients' troubles. The ways in which they accomplish this are infused not only with false expectations of medical science, but also with cultural assumptions about gender.

Gendered Medical Language: Women's Bodies as Fragmented and Degraded

When the women I spoke with discovered that their "minor" implant-related complications could have been signs of serious trouble, they found fault with their physicians for "intentionally" withholding information from them. However, blaming physicians ignores the complex process through which prevailing beliefs about medical science interact with cultural assumptions about gender, shaping the ways in which physicians have responded to women's problems with implants. In particular, the language physicians used to divert attention away from the uncertainty of women's problems is infused with images of failed, degraded, and fragmented female bodies.

The dominant medical perspective in Western culture is predicated on the belief that knowledge about health and illness is obtainable through scientific inquiry. "Good" science is presumed to be objective and value-free—the more detached the investigator is from the object of study, the closer she or he will be able to arrive at the "truth." Deborah Gordon explains, "The western philosophic and scientific traditions have long assumed that detachment provides the purest window to truth. . . . To arrive at real knowledge we must alter ourselves—move back, distance ourselves from values, local bias, and particular interest by taking a universal standpoint, one which is disengaged from everyday life."[6] This distancing from daily life understandings and experiences is a goal of medical practice. Physicians generally approach sickness as a distinctly biological phenomenon, or "an autonomous entity, defined by standard universal criteria, isolated from the lives and experiences of patients."[7] In this way, "the biological model strips away social contexts of meaning."[8]

Technological advances and increases in specialization have contributed to the tendency of medical practitioners to ignore the emotions and personal life experiences that affect how individuals think about themselves, as well as how they think about health and illness. These developments have permitted physicians to focus on specific anatomical parts or single bodily processes to improve their understanding of disease etiologies. However, they have also contributed to the perception of the human body as "a machine without a mind or soul."[9] For example, focusing on the impact of reproductive technologies on medical practice, Emily Martin notes, "Human eggs, sperm and embryos can now be moved from body to body or out of and back into the same female body. The organic unity of fetus and mother can no longer be assumed, and all these newly fragmented parts can now be subjected to market forces, ordered, produced, bought, and sold."[10]

Medical science has treated both male and female bodies as if consisting of isolated, mechanical parts to be manipulated and cured. Nevertheless, feminist scholars argue that since women historically have been alienated from the production of medical and scientific knowledge, the content of medical science has been based on a "male-biased model of human nature and social reality."[11] Researchers and scholars have demonstrated this bias in a number of ways. For instance, the biologist Anne Fausto-Sterling is widely known for her research that calls into question "scientific" interpretations of biologically based sex differences.[12] Fausto-Sterling suggests that since Western medical science traditionally has appointed the male reproductive life cycle as "normal," any aspect of female reproduction that deviates from the male's has been viewed as "abnormal."[13] Consequently, a wide range of normal, female bodily processes, including menopause and menstruation, have been defined by medical and scientific experts as disease states.

Similarly, Alexandra Dundas Todd asserts that the dominant medical perspective has led to "a legacy of women's bodies being defined, by the virtue of their very existence, as [diseased and] deviant." [14]

Emily Martin's cultural analysis of reproduction further demonstrates a male-dominated perspective in medical science. [15] In particular, Martin shows how metaphors of economic mass production have informed scientific descriptions of female bodies within medical textbooks. These descriptions are replete with images of failed functions, deprivation, and decline. For instance, one text depicts menstruation as follows: "The fall in blood progesterone and estrogen 'deprives' the 'highly developed endometrial lining of its hormonal support,' 'constriction' of blood vessels leads to a 'diminished' supply of oxygen and nutrients, and finally 'disintegration starts, the entire lining begins to slough, and the menstrual flow begins.'" [16] Susan Bell found similar imagery in scientific papers on menopause, which explained this natural bodily process in terms of a "deficiency disease." [17] In short, the exclusion of women in the production of medical and scientific knowledge has perpetuated the view that female bodies are not only machines consisting of fragmented parts to be manipulated by medical mechanics, but also inherently "flawed" and "defective."

The cultural perception of women's bodies as inherently diseased, combined with the societal reliance on medical technology to "treat" and "cure" women's perceived problems, has led physicians to attribute blame to women's bodies when medical interventions fail. Bell's analysis of an interview with a woman she calls "Sarah" illustrates this point. [18] Sarah's prenatal exposure to diethylstilbestrol (DES) prevented her from carrying her pregnancy to term. [19] Nevertheless, her physician attributed her miscarriage to her "incompetent cervix"—a term that "blames the victim for the problem." [20]

My respondents' descriptions of their physicians' responses to their ruptured and encapsulated breast implants were replete with similar language. For instance, when Karen's breasts hardened after receiving implants, her surgeon implied that her body was at fault—not her implants; she reported, "When I began to experience the hardening, the surgeon made it seem as if there was something wrong with my body. You know, almost as if, 'Oh you are having such and such.' Sort of like, 'Well this is what happens and your body is just reacting this way'— instead of saying, 'There is something wrong with the implant.' You know, there was no talk of this."

In Jane's case, her physician not only blamed her body for her implant-related complication but, in so doing, disregarded the potential seriousness of her problem. After Jane returned home from an appointment for her annual mammogram, she received a phone call from her primary care physician. The purpose of his call was to inform Jane that one of her implants had ruptured:

> He calls me up on the phone and he says, "Well, it looks like you sprung a leak."
>> I said, "Excuse me, who is this?"
>> And he says, "This is Dr. Jones."
>> And I said, "Sprung a leak? What are you talking about?"
>> And he goes, "Your mammogram. You have breast implants don't you?"

Cultural assumptions about female bodies as inherently "flawed" pervade the logic that guides this description of Jane's problem: Jane's implant did not "spring a leak"—her own body did. Such a description not only attributes blame to Jane's body, but it also conveys the hierarchical image of the female body as a machine to be tinkered with and mechanically manipulated by medical experts. Moreover, by focusing solely on the results of her mammogram, Jane's physician treated her body as if it were separate and detached from her self. Consequently, he failed to consider how Jane might react to the discovery that her implant had ruptured and that she would need additional surgery to remove it. In response, Jane was angry and upset.

Soon after her conversation with this physician, Jane visited her plastic surgeon and was reassured. He explained that he could easily "fix" her problem by removing both of her implants and replacing them with new and improved versions of these devices. When Jane asked this doctor if she should be concerned about the silicone from the ruptured implant, he assured her again saying, "Oh, that is no big deal. It comes right out." However, what Jane had thought would be a forty-five-minute procedure to replace her damaged implants turned into a three-and-a-half-hour surgery—Jane's plastic surgeon removed not only her implants but also surrounding breast tissue that was contaminated with silicone. When Jane awakened from her surgery and asked her doctor why it had taken so long and why she was in so much pain, he replied, "Well, I did a lot of work on you." Again, the mechanical metaphor (i.e., doing "work" on a body as if it were a machine), detaches feelings and emotions from physical bodies, while concealing the potential seriousness of women's implant-related problems.

Misdiagnosing Women's Symptoms: "If It's Not in Your Body, It Must Be in Your Head"

The women I interviewed were angry at their physicians not only for treating their ruptured and encapsulated implants as minor and common complications, but also for failing to take seriously the strange progression of symptoms they began experiencing after receiving implants. In particular, the majority of women I interviewed reported that when they visited their physicians with autoimmune symptoms such as aching joints, rashes, hair loss, and fatigue, their doctors minimized these problems by relegating them to the realms of either reproductive or psychological complaints. For instance, as Sheila's health slowly began to deteriorate several years following her plastic surgery, she went to many different medical specialists hoping to find an explanation for the wide range of symptoms she was experiencing. Instead, she said that practically every physician she visited was unable to find a medical diagnosis to account for her worsening health. In effect, her doctors simply assumed that Sheila's problems must either be emotionally based or stem from some other "female" condition.

Sheila received her implants in 1973 at the age of twenty-nine. Ten years later she began experiencing health problems. In particular, she had sore throats and felt feverish and achy nearly one week out of every month. Since these symptoms usually occurred during the time she was menstruating, Sheila logically assumed that they were related to her reproductive cycle. Thus, she scheduled an appointment with her gynecologist. Sheila visited this doctor, who diagnosed her condition as "bad PMS." Having no reason to doubt her physician's medical expertise, Sheila accepted this diagnosis and went about her daily life trying to ignore her symptoms. However, her health increasingly deteriorated over the next few years. Sheila not only felt sick during the days around her period, but for a couple of weeks out of every month. Moreover, as her old health problems worsened, new ones began to emerge—her extreme fatigue and sore throats were now accompanied with frequent dizziness, disorientation, and aching joints. Sheila explained that some days her symptoms were so debilitating that she could barely get out of bed in the morning to go to work—she had to call in sick more and more frequently. Concerned and afraid, she returned to her gynecologist, explaining, "My symptoms are interfering with my work—I have been taking two to three days off every month." Nevertheless, her doctor continued to respond by telling her, "It's bad PMS."

In 1991, Sheila said that she felt so sick, frustrated, and "fed up," that she decided to switch to a different gynecologist. After describing her symptoms to him, he referred her to an endocrinologist to check for a potential "hormonal imbalance." However, even this specialist was unable to find anything physically wrong with Sheila because all of her tests came back "normal." Sheila explained, "Everything—my hormone levels, my estrogen level, everything was fine." Unable to attribute her ailments to any known hormonal or reproductive disorder, this doctor told Sheila that she ought to consider the possibility that her problems were emotionally based and recommended that she see a psychiatrist.

Sheila resisted believing that her troubles stemmed from a psychological problem and decided to visit another specialist (a neurologist), hoping to find some explanation that would account for her worsening symptoms. At this point, Sheila said that she was so disoriented at times that she was having difficulty responding to people when they spoke to her. Sometimes she could barely make sense of what they were saying: "It was like people were talking a different language to me." Moreover, she was so fatigued that she was unable to drive her car and considered quitting her job. When she reported these symptoms to her neurologist, he examined her and arranged for her to have a brain scan. However, again, the results of Sheila's tests came back "normal." Just as Sheila's endocrinologist relegated her problems to the realm of emotional complaints when he was unable to come up with a medical diagnosis for her, so, too, did her neurologist. Sheila explained, "He said to me, 'You are depressed. You need to go to a psychiatrist. You have all of the symptoms of depression.'" Feeling helpless and hopeless, Sheila responded to this doctor by saying, "If I am depressed, it is because I am sick and I would like to know what is wrong with me. But I am not a depressed person. I mean, how can I be a depressed person and work fifteen hours a day and take care of two kids and run a house? You don't know me. This is not how I am." Despite Sheila's plea, her physician wrote in his patient evaluation that she was depressed and needed psychiatric care. Sheila's fiancé also began to believe that her problems were all in her head, saying to her, "Maybe you are depressed and you just don't know it." Sheila described the range of emotions she felt after realizing that even her closest companion was unable to validate her troubles: "It is really bad to really feel that sick . . . when you can't get help and nobody knows what is wrong with you. You feel like you are on a cliff and you are hanging on and nobody is grabbing your hand. And when they say, 'Go to a psychiatrist,' they are pushing you off the cliff."

After visiting many more doctors who denied the existence of her health problems, Sheila eventually found a primary care physician who diagnosed her with chronic fatigue syndrome and a number of other autoimmune-related conditions. This physician also asked Sheila to consider the possibility that her poor health might be related to her implants. By now, Sheila had heard news reports about a possible link between breast implants and immunological and rheumatic disorders and began to suspect that her own implants were contributing to her problems. In 1993, when Sheila went for her annual mammogram, her radiologist found that both of her implants had ruptured. A pathology report confirmed that silicone had migrated into her breast tissue and that her body was showing a reaction to it. Given this information, Sheila was certain that her history of strange symptoms was directly related to her breast implants.

Sheila's description of her encounters with physicians sounds similar to the experiences of other women I interviewed who claimed that their doctors minimized the health problems they experienced after receiving breast implants. Abby, who runs a support group for women with breast implants, commented, "Everyone [in our group] was all feeling the same way, but when we went to the doctors, we were told that you are going through menopause or you need to see a psychiatrist. They just don't associate implants with the sickness we have." Abby said that her doctors, too, misdiagnosed her implant-related symptoms as signs of early menopause.

Frances also reported that her doctors did not take her health problems seriously. She believed that her implants might be related to her feeling sick all the time, but every time she mentioned "silicone" to her doctors, "they either had no response or they look at you like you are a fifty-year-old woman going through the change." Frances explained that after she mentioned to one of her doctors that she was experiencing sleeplessness, chronic fatigue, and aching joints, he wrote in her chart that she was exhibiting "severe anxiety attacks," telling her she needed psychological counseling.

Other women also commented that their doctors relegated their symptoms to the realm of emotional complaints. Leslie said that one of her doctors felt that a prescription of Prozac would solve all of her "implant-related" troubles. And, after Jenna expressed her concerns and fears about her breast implants to her rheumatologist, he recommended that she visit a psychiatrist. Jenna followed his suggestion, thinking that counseling might help alleviate some of her anxiety. However, when she explained to her psychiatrist that she was afraid that her implants had ruptured, he, too, dismissed her concerns, saying, "I do not think that it is your implants that are exploding, I think it is your life that is exploding!"

The descriptions of medical mistreatment experienced by the women I interviewed resonate with social science research that suggests that women patients, in general, are not taken seriously, and are viewed as "overemotional," "neurotic," "difficult," and unable to understand complicated medical explanations.[21] Social historians suggest that these assumptions originated in the nineteenth century and have been perpetuated through medical discourse ever since. Barbara Ehrenreich and Deirdre English, for example, assert that the rise of medical experts during this time period increasingly led to the construction of "femininity" as a disease.[22] In order to ensure their growing profession and sustain the sexual division of labor at the brink of industrial growth, medical men increasingly exerted control over women's lives, claiming that the instability of their reproductive cycles made them unfit for wider social roles. In the latter half of the 1800s young women were discouraged from partaking in educational pursuits that would draw them away from (and thus damage) their reproductive organs. During the same time, physicians routinely prescribed "a renewed commitment to asexual domesticity" to older women experiencing "menopausal disease" who were violating their "feminine" role by engaging in sexual intercourse.[23] In fact, by the late nineteenth century, gynecologists and psychologists ascribed nearly all female diseases to reproductive malfunctions, which interfered with women's "sexual, emotional, and rational control."[24] Subsequently, it was not uncommon for doctors to prescribe sexual surgery (i.e., the removal of a woman's clitoris or ovaries) as a means of "curing" female insanity, neurosis, abnormal menstruation, and any other condition relevant to female behavior.[25]

Although twentieth-century medicine has abandoned nineteenth-century methods and procedures used to treat "female" maladies, feminist scholars assert that women's lives continue to be vulnerable to the damaging consequences of medicalization. For example, Sheryl Ruzek suggests that the medicalization of pregnancy and childbirth continues to increase the likelihood that women will suffer the iatrogenic effects of medical practices, devices, and drugs.[26] A prime example of this is the trend toward more cesarean births, which places childbirth exclusively in the hands of physicians, while increasing the risk of infection.[27] In addition to such practices, recent medical innovations developed solely for women have been promoted with claims of safety and efficacy that have far outstripped reality.[28] For instance, along with breast implants, the Dalkon Shield (an intrauterine device marketed in the early 1970s), the first birth control pill, and the synthetic hormone DES have all been associated with numerous dangerous side effects.[29]

Medical labels that define women's natural bodily and physiological functions as diseased states have not only perpetuated the use of dangerous drugs and devices, but have also contributed to perceived behavioral differences between men and women. An example illustrating this point is the wide acceptance of premenstrual syndrome as a medical diagnosis for "female" irritability, depression, and mood swings.[30] The perception of women as overemotional by virtue of the "instability" of their hormonal and reproductive cycles may negatively affect women's lives, since it perpetuates and reinforces the notion that they are inherently unequipped to handle roles of leadership and responsibility.[31]

Given the history of the relationship between women and medicine, it is not surprising that many of the women I met believed that their status as "female patient" hindered any chance they had at finding medical validation for their troubles. Eve explained, "I think all of my physicians just pooh-poohed everything about implants. And, especially as a woman, you walk in there and you are automatically—and if you have a male physician you are at an even greater disadvantage because when you come in and you are upset about something, they automatically assume that it's the wrong time of the month or you are just an emotional woman." Some women reported that even physicians who were women treated their implant-related troubles as signs of less serious "female" conditions.[32] This finding resonates with work of other researchers who have found that men and women doctors do not differ in their evaluations of patients' complaints, and that even though women may begin their medical training with a more humanistic and nurturing perspective, by the time they are practicing, their attitudes resemble those of men. In other words, they are less caring and less patient-oriented.[33]

The women I interviewed were angry and disillusioned with medical care, claiming that their doctors used their professional authority to minimize their troubles and "put them in their place" to protect their reputations. However, such an explanation fails to take into account how cultural assumptions about gender interact with predominating beliefs about medical science, continually creating tensions between doctors and their female patients. For example, Sheila's physicians' responses to her symptoms illustrate how the cultural assumption that women are inherently overemotional interacts with the dominant medical belief that disease causation can be understood in a context where bodies are fragmented into isolated parts to be cured. Even though Sheila's symptoms sounded nearly identical to those experienced by other women I interviewed who were diagnosed with chronic fatigue syndrome and other immunological disorders, Sheila had difficulty finding a physician who was able to make sense of all of her physical troubles. Instead, when Sheila approached each of them with her symptoms, they ruled out only the conditions and diseases that they were equipped to understand within their fields of specialization—her gynecologist believed Sheila had a reproductive problem, her endocrinologist checked for a hormonal imbalance, and her neurologist ordered a brain scan hoping to understand why she was experiencing cognitive difficulties. The inability of these doctors to understand Sheila's health troubles outside the narrow scope of their own medical specialties resulted in their belief that Sheila's problem must be psychological, not physical.

After Eleanor had received breast implants and began experiencing numerous symptoms, she, too, was under the care of many different doctors, yet none of them linked her problems to her implants: "Here is an immunologist, here is an internist, here is a plastic surgeon—all three, and I was also under the care of the urologist—he was still looking at me. A lot of specialized people looking at one little thing and not looking at the whole picture. Everyone kept everything so separate." In this comment, Eleanor identifies a distinction between modern medicine, which is characterized by the tendency of medical specialists to focus on separate physiological processes, and a more holistic approach toward health care (that views the "whole picture"). Although Eleanor implicitly linked the inability of her physicians to acknowledge a potential relationship between her implants and her worsening health to the structure of modern medicine, she, nevertheless, attributed blame to her individual doctors: "You know, in hindsight, how could nobody even say, 'Gee, Eleanor just had her breasts reconstructed with implants'—that was never written in these doctors' reports. They could have written that I had just had surgery and that possibly my body was having an autoimmune reaction. You know—something! Why wasn't there a connection made?"

Responses to the Scientific Evidence

For Eleanor and other women I spoke with, the relationship between their exposure to silicone and their worsening health seemed all too obvious for their physicians to miss. Yet, at the same time, epidemiological and scientific studies have consistently found no evidence of a significant relationship between implants and disease. For example, the results of the Mayo Clinic study on implant-related risk "do not support an association between breast implants and connective-tissue diseases or other disorders that were studied."[34] Similarly, every investigation on the long-term health effects of silicone breast implants presented in a recent volume of the *Journal of Clinical Epidemiology* found no evidence of an increased risk among implant recipients of breast carcinoma,[35] soft-tissue carcinoma,[36] breast cancer,[37] systemic sclerosis,[38] and rheumatoid arthritis or other diffuse connective-tissue disease.[39]

In order to explain the contradiction between the results of these studies and anecdotal evidence that suggests a link between illness and breast implants, the women I interviewed alluded to a political bias in the production of scientific knowledge. Some women specifically focused on the Mayo Clinic study as an example of how the medical and scientific communities conspire to keep their troubles with implants silent. In the early 1990s, the number of women who believed they had been harmed by breast implants had escalated to such an extent that a global settlement had been proposed in order to determine which implant recipients would be reimbursed based on the problems they had experienced. The Mayo Clinic study had received a tremendous amount of media attention since not only was it published in a highly reputable medical journal (the *New England Journal of Medicine*), but also it appeared in print the day before women with implants had to decide whether or not to participate in this settlement. Thus, women interpreted the timing and placement of the paper as a strategic move on the part of plastic surgeons to scare implant recipients away from pursuing litigation, or to perpetuate the belief that those who joined the class action suit were simply "jumping on the bandwagon."

Other women I interviewed based their criticisms of "scientific" studies that found no evidence of a relationship between implants and disease on the grounds that the research was either funded by plastic surgeons associations or implant manufacturers,[40] or was conducted by researchers who were consultants to law firms representing implant manufacturers in lawsuits brought by women who believed they had been harmed by the devices.[41] Recognizing these possible biases, Paula exclaimed, "All the studies [on implant-related risk] that are being done should not be funded by the manufacturers and plastic surgeons—they shouldn't be paying for it! Maybe the government should be putting in the money so that no strings are attached, and so that researchers can really study the *women* and not base their research on looking at their old records and seeing what their records say, because the records are false or inaccurate half the time." This remark is directed, again, at the Mayo Clinic study. The study was based on a comparative analysis of 749 medical records of women who had breast implants, and 1,498 who were not implanted with these devices. Paula's criticism implies that research based solely on medical records, rather than on interviews with patients, may be entirely futile since physicians tend to record only information they view as "medically relevant," and not based on women's own descriptions of how they feel. This criticism also is discussed in the sociological literature. For instance, Harold Garfinkle suggests that physicians' medical records are inconsistent and lack detail about patients' daily life experiences.[42] Rebecca's description of her plastic surgeon's response to the pain she was experiencing in her chest, arms, and ribs after receiving implants further illustrates this possibility:

Nobody really seemed to be concerned about anything—particularly the plastic surgeon, never. I don't think he ever even wrote down—you know, we would discuss it, but I never saw him write down that I was having any pains. . . . And, when I described this, I remember vividly his saying to me on several occasions, "No one else has ever complained of that." Or, "I haven't heard that problem." And, it would always—I would leave his office and I would always ask myself, "How can he say that? He isn't even writing down what I'm saying. So, if he's not documenting what I'm saying, then there's no evidence that anyone has had any problems [laughs] because it's just not there.

The predominating belief in Western culture is that knowledge based on scientific "facts" is more accurate and precise than knowledge based on life experiences and personal feelings. However, the ways in which some of the women I interviewed interpreted the scientific evidence on implant-related risk implicitly suggests that even when knowledge has been acquired through rigorous and systematic study (or, guided by "scientific rationality"), it is nevertheless shaped by larger political and economic contexts. Evelyn Fox Keller similarly asserts that scientific knowledge is never objective, but inescapably value-laden, since it is always "shaped by our choices—first, of what to seek representations *of*, and second, of what to seek representations *for.*"[43] Many of my respondents believe that their physicians resisted acknowledging a possible link between implants and disease because they were afraid of losing profits and jeopardizing their professional reputations. In effect, they preferred to rely on "biased" scientific evidence that consistently reported that implants are safe, rather than giving credibility to women's reports of their worsening physical symptoms. Perceived as medically irrelevant, these symptoms were never recorded in women's medical evaluations and, therefore, according to certain studies, never even existed.

The Emergence of New Scientific Evidence: Are Breast Implants Now "Safe"?

After I finished conducting my initial interviews with women in 1994, new studies and publications began to emerge that further addressed the possible dangers of silicone breast implants. For instance, a 1996 study conducted by researchers from Boston's Brigham and Women's Hospital and the Harvard Schools of Medicine and Public Health examined the relationship between breast implants and various forms of connective-tissue diseases. Rather than depend on patient evaluations, the study used self-reports from a large sample of over 400,000 female health professionals as data.[44] This research which, to date, is the largest investigation of the health effects of breast implants, has stimulated even further debate over whether implants pose a threat to women's health. Although the authors of the study did find a small increased risk of connective-tissue diseases among breast implant recipients, they also concluded that their results "provide reassuring evidence against a large hazard of breast implants on connective-tissue diseases."[45] The *Boston*

Globe quoted one epidemiologist who remarked, "When I saw the results [of this study], I said 'Oh, boy, it's going to be interpreted in whatever way people want to interpret it.'"[46] Indeed, the *New York Times* reported that a week before the study was published, implant manufacturers were already using it as evidence that breast implants were safe. Now that the study has been published, lawyers representing women in lawsuits against these manufacturers are using the same study as evidence that implants cause disease.[47]

Consumer advocacy groups supporting women who believe they have been harmed by implants have also commented on the study. For instance, Sidney Wolfe, the director of Public Citizen in Washington, D.C., asserts that the Brigham and Women's study, as well as other epidemiological investigations on the long-term health effects of breast implants, has come to the conclusion that implants do not pose a significant threat to women's health, because they all have focused on classical forms of immunological disorders or connective tissue diseases. Women with breast implants, on the other hand, seem to have atypical forms of these illnesses.[48] The authors of the Brigham and Women's retrospective cohort study, themselves, state, "We did not assess the occurrence of atypical connective-tissue diseases or syndromes (such as fibromyalgia or chronic fatigue syndrome) or subjective symptoms (such as chronic fatigue or arthralgia). . . . It is difficult to study any relation of breast implants with these atypical diseases or syndromes, because currently these conditions possess no validated classification criteria."[49] In other words, the diagnostic technology has not been developed to test for these new patterns or forms of diseases.

Frank Vasey, a rheumatologist who has seen many cases of women with breast implants experiencing autoimmune-type symptoms, suggests that while implant recipients do not test positive for diseases such as rheumatoid arthritis, lupus, and scleroderma, their symptoms are, nevertheless, consistent with those characterized by these conditions. In fact, many of the women I interviewed who were experiencing chronic fatigue, general achiness, hair loss, and a variety of other symptoms explained that their physicians consistently tested them for immunological disorders and connective-tissue diseases; however, the results of these tests almost always came back "normal." Abby, for instance, remarked, "When you go to the doctor and get blood work taken, sometimes your range may not fall within the expected norm of the diseases. So, you go away—you know that you are sick, but the blood work doesn't come up that you are sick." Similarly, Lorraine explained, "No one can seem to put their finger on what is causing my symptoms. Some doctors think I may have arthritis, so they do the test. I don't have arthritis, but I have aches around my joints, and there are some mornings I can get up and I can hardly walk and bend." Vasey suggests that women with implants may be experiencing a new form of illness he refers to as "silicone disease." Single lab tests can not confirm the presence of this illness because the technology does not currently exist.[50] As a result, "physicians have not been able to identify the disease in their patients, and therefore have instituted a long chain of blind testing and trial medications."[51] Or, as many of my respondents believe, when physicians are unable to attribute their patients' symptoms to any known medical condition, they relegate them to the realms of reproductive malfunctions or emotional problems.

Frank Vasey is not the first to question modern medicine's ability to recognize and treat new forms of disease. For instance, Marc Lappé, a pathologist whose laboratory research supports a connection between silicone and autoimmune disease,[52] suggests that the dominant medical perspective in our culture fails to take into account the interplay between the natural world and human adaptations to it. In effect, modern medicine provides merely snapshots of disease—"glimpses of illnesses frozen in time and space. . . . This tendency to abstract dynamic, evolving processes into discrete moments, generates an understandable lack of appreciation of what [diseases and epidemics] came before and what will come after."[53] Moreover, it has led to a "special blindness to the natural forces that have shaped human disease."[54] A prime example of this shortsightedness is reflected in social science literature that criticizes physicians and scientists for their lack of familiarity with the health problems that may result from exposure to environmental hazards and contaminated waste sites.[55] Similarly, some of the women I interviewed found fault with their physicians for relying solely on diagnostic testing and scientific "facts" presented in prestigious medical journals to arrive at a conclusion about a relationship between breast implants and disease. Sheila commented:

> It has been my experience that if [disease causation] is not black and white— and if it is not presented in an article in a prominent medical journal, then [according to physicians] the disease doesn't exist. . . . There are so many new diseases out there—like, all these new bacteria and viruses that doctors don't know about. And, they don't have the tests for them. The problem with this

whole silicone issue is that they have no tests. For instance, there is no blood test yet to see if there is silicone traveling around in your body—that would clear up questions around that issue real fast—but they simply don't have the test.

Brenda also believes that women with implants are experiencing a "new disease" that the medical community has failed to recognize: "Medical science and the medical community are two different groups. The science aspect to this debate over implants will perhaps not marry the medical community for another ten years. . . . If you read up on the information on breast implants, they only began questioning the safety of these devices within the past ten years. We are experiencing a new disease. Now, what is causing this disease? I guarantee down the road, the science will catch up with this and they will make a connection with implants." Comparing their own experiences with diagnostic testing to physicians' inability to recognize new patterns or forms of disease allowed Sheila and Brenda to acknowledge the possibility that medical knowledge is never complete, but always uncertain and continuously evolving. According to these women, a cause-and-effect relationship between implants and disease has yet to be determined since science has not found a way of understanding and diagnosing new patterns of "silicone-related" illnesses.[56]

In her recent book *Science on Trial: The Clash of Medical Evidence and the Law in the Breast Implant Case*, Marcia Angell, the executive editor of the *New England Journal of Medicine*, takes a stance on breast implants that diverges from views expressed by most of the women I interviewed, as well as clinicians and researchers such as Frank Vasey and Marc Lappé.[57] Relying solely on epidemiological studies to determine whether a causal relationship between implants and disease exists, Angell asserts that "any connection between implants and connective tissue disease is likely to be very weak, at most, since several good studies have failed to detect it."[58]

In light of the most recent scientific evidence, Angell argues that the controversy over breast implants is less about women experiencing actual illnesses than it is about greedy plaintiff attorneys relying on speculative theories and anecdotal evidence in order to win exorbitant awards in breast implant litigation. Angell does not deny the possibility that some women with implants may experience a variety of symptoms such as insomnia, muscle aches, and fatigue; but, rather than attribute these symptoms to women's implants, she dismisses them as "ordinary symptoms of life." [59] According to Angell, the FDA's 1992 decision to restrict the use of breast implants and the media hype about the dangers of these devices that followed have caused unnecessary alarm among implant recipients, magnifying their perceived health troubles. She explains, "When people are afraid that they might have a serious disease, they often feel worse than they would if they had no such concerns." [60] Dismissing women's complaints as normal symptoms of everyday life and relying completely on scientific evidence for the "truth" about breast implants, Angell views the large number of personal-injury suits against implant manufacturers as a reflection of society's failure to understand and accept the collective opinion of professional experts who derive knowledge from "careful scientific research" and "unbiased interpretation of the results." [61]

Angell's stance on the breast implant debate resonates with views expressed in recent media reports. For instance, a 1995 *New York Times* article titled "Implant Lawsuits Create a Medical Rush to Cash In," implies that the increasing number of women claiming they have been injured by their implants simply reflects the actions of greedy plaintiffs and their attorneys. [62] A month after this report, the *Chicago Tribune* and the *New York Times* reported on the American College of Rheumatology's stance that silicone breast implants do not lead to an increased risk of connective-tissue or rheumatic disease. [63] The college condemned plaintiff attorneys handling implant litigation for harassing scientists and urged the FDA and courts to stop giving credence to anecdotal evidence that implants lead to disease. Editors of the *Los Angeles Times* expressed a similar view, asserting that Dow Corning and other implant manufacturers were forced into a settlement because "tort lawyers have managed to use anecdotal evidence . . . to persuade juries that there is a causative link [between implants and disease]." [64] More recently, journalists reported on a 1996 federal court ruling that prevents plaintiff lawyers from introducing evidence that implants cause disease. [65] The decision was made after court-appointed experts determined that the evidence was "not scientifically valid."

Although epidemiological evidence, to date, suggests that breast implants do not lead to autoimmune diseases, a 1997 study conducted by Mayo Clinic researchers and published in the *New England Journal of Medicine* indicates that the devices can cause local complications that are serious enough to require additional surgery. [66] Thomas Burton of the *Wall Street Journal* reported that the results of this study "could shift the debate over silicone away from immune-system illnesses and toward such chest-area ailments as abnormal tissue growth and chronic pain."[67] A recent news segment on *Prime Time Live* provides evidence of this shift in focus.[68] The segment was about a clinical trial under way for breast implants filled with soybean oil—a potentially safer alternative to the silicone-gel-filled devices. While the show conveyed the message that silicone breast implants have bad side effects, the only dangers addressed were capsular contracture, ruptures, and other localized complications—there was no mention of the possibility that these implants can lead to disabling autoimmune diseases. Thus, while the most recent epidemiological study on implant-related risk may validate some women's experiences, it may minimize the experiences of others who have disabling symptoms apart from, or in addition to, various local complications.

Women's Responses to the Continuing Debate

While breast implants continue to receive a great deal of media attention, the information disseminated to the public over the past three years reflects a trend toward minimizing the side effects associated with these devices. In order to get a sense of how implant recipients were responding to this trend, I conducted follow-up interviews with six women who had expressed diverging views on the breast implant controversy during my initial interviews with them.[69] In 1994, Tracy, Sheila, and Eve were all convinced that there was a relationship between implants and disease; Lorraine and Barbara suspected that their health problems might be caused by their implants, but did not feel they had enough information to confirm this belief; and Maureen strongly believed that implants were "safe," and that women who believed otherwise were simply "jumping on the band wagon." In addition to conducting these interviews, I also was able to gain insights into how women were responding to recent media reports and scientific studies by reading newspaper commentaries and online discussion groups and message boards for women with breast implants I accessed through the Internet.[70]

Despite scientific evidence and media accounts that suggest that the relationship between breast implants and disease is "not significant," the women in my follow-up study who had experienced a variety of vague and ambiguous symptoms when I first interviewed them were convinced more than ever that their breast implants were contributing to their worsening health. Sheila, who still experiences aching joints and flulike symptoms, but whose tests continue to come back "normal," commented, "I am completely convinced that my symptoms are related to my implants. . . . I know that a lot of women deteriorated and broke down because they gave in to the whole thing and believed what the doctors and media was telling them, but not me."

Similarly, Eve whose aching joints, chronic fatigue, and hair loss subsided after having her silicone breast implants were removed a year and a half ago, remarked, "I think that the studies that have come out are very narrow-based. I am sure there are some women out there who rely on these studies and want to bury their heads in the sand and say, 'I am fine.' But, there isn't anybody in the world that can sit in front of me and tell me my implants did not cause what was wrong with me." And, Tracy, who started her own support network for women with breast implants, commented, "A lot of women with breast implants did not have preexisting medical conditions prior to having implants. And, now the scientific literature is trying to come up with the idea that the symptoms we now experience are because we are getting older, or have had a bad marriage, or are premenstrual—the studies are biased."

Even Lorraine and Barbara, the two women I spoke to who had been reluctant to acknowledge the possibility that their health problems were related to their breast implants, were now willing to make this connection. Lorraine, who had her breast implants removed a year ago, explained, "I still have all kinds of symptoms that no one can put their finger on. They could very well be related to middle age. But my symptoms have lessened since the implants were removed. . . . I just know that I was not feeling well with them, and I do feel somewhat better now." Barbara, whose symptoms have worsened over the course of the past two years, just learned that one of her breast implants is ruptured. She, too, now believes the devices are contributing to her poor health and is in the process of searching for a plastic surgeon who will remove them.

Many of the views about breast implants expressed by the women I interviewed are shared by women who participate in online discussions over the Internet. For instance, in response to the most recent Mayo Clinic study, one implant recipient writes: "The Mayo clinic has just perpetrated an unforgivable crime on the medical and scientific world by publishing their most recent study on 'local complications' of silicone breast implants, in which they FORGET to say that their prior study of 'classical' connective tissue disease and silicone breast implants DID NOT EXAMINE THE RISK of 'non-classical' diseases. . . . That proper epidemiological studies have not been done is NOT PROOF that there is no problem."[71] Commentaries in newspapers written by women with implants uncover similar sentiments of anger and outrage directed at scientific researchers, the medical community, implant manufacturers, and the media for perpetuating the "myth" that implants are "safe." In a recent issue of the *Columbia Daily Tribune*, a leader of a support group for women with breast implants remarks, "We feel that we have been 'raped' by the media which . . . has swallowed the manufacturers' line that we are victims of some sort of medical and legal hoax."[72]

While the majority of women who publicly voice their opinions about breast implants are convinced of a causal relationship between implants and disease, a few women express an opposing point of view. For instance, Marilyn Lloyd, a former member of Congress from Tennessee who received silicone breast implants following a mastectomy, takes Marcia Angell's side on the implant debate. In a commentary printed in the *Chicago Tribune*, she writes: "Opponents of breast implants have no good scientific evidence. Instead they count on jurors' compassion for women who are all ill (or believe they are) and disdain for big corporations who made the devices. . . . It seems to be that what's driving the implant scare is mainly money. Lawyers are in a feeding frenzy over the prospect of huge jury awards or out-of-court-settlements."[73] Another woman whose commentary appeared in a more recent issue of the *Chicago Tribune* also bases her knowledge about breast implants on the scientific evidence: "I know 20 major studies, at institutions ranging from the Harvard School of medicine to the Mayo Clinic and Johns Hopkins have failed to find any connection between breast implants and a large increased risk of disease trial lawyers attribute to them." Although this woman's implant had ruptured, she takes pride in not "succumb[ing] to the fear-mongering of lawyers," further stating that women "have a right to legal recourse, but only if their claims are supported by fact."[74] Women who rely on the scientific evidence for the "facts" about breast implants also express their views over the Internet. For instance, one woman posts a message announcing that she is "thrilled" with her new saline breast implants. She further comments, "I know that saline implants have the silicone shell . . . but, the last I heard, there was still NO medical proof linking silicone to any of the reported medical problems."[75] During my second interview with Maureen, she, too, expressed the view that breast implants were safe until science proved them otherwise. Maureen was so convinced by recent studies that there is no connection between autoimmune diseases and implants that she decided to undergo surgery to replace her saline implant with a silicone one, feeling that the silicone would look and feel more natural.

Recent books, media reports, and scientific studies all convey the message that the controversy over silicone breast implants, to a certain extent, is settled—the devices do not lead to disabling autoimmune diseases. However, evidence from my follow-up study suggests that this debate is far from over in the minds of implant recipients themselves. While some women continue to place their trust in the scientific evidence and in doctors who tell them they are "fine," others have chosen to break away from the dominant medical perspective that reinforced their physicians' tendency to minimize their implant-related experiences. As I have demonstrated throughout this chapter, reliance on this dominant perspective led many physicians to base their evaluations of women's troubles on diagnostic tests and scientific studies, rather than on women's own descriptions of their symptoms and concerns. This inevitably led these doctors to minimize women's implant-related complications, misdiagnose their symptoms, and perpetuate the view that women's *real* troubles were all in their heads, not in their bodies.

Learning how to evaluate and scrutinize the scientific evidence on implant-related risk, and recognizing the fallibility of medical knowledge, most of the women who participated in my study no longer relied on the voice of medical science to determine whether their symptoms were real; instead, they chose to listen to an inner voice that shaped their knowledge about health, illness, and disease causation.

7

Listening to an Inner Voice

*A*lthough many women with breast implants may go about their daily lives without any implant-related symptoms and concerns, these women did not represent the majority of women who participated in this study. In fact, 85 percent of the forty women I interviewed reported experiencing a variety of health problems they believed to be associated with their implants, and 90 percent were terribly concerned that their breast implants would inevitably lead either to new health problems or worsening conditions. Considering these high proportions, it is not surprising that many of the women I spoke with blame the individuals and institutions that were involved in providing them with a potentially dangerous medical device.

While some of the women I interviewed continued to blame themselves for having agreed to undergo surgery simply to feel more "feminine" or more "whole," many others had moved away from feeling responsible for their troubles. Turning their emotions outwards, they directed blame at the specific agencies, industries, or individuals responsible for the inadequate regulation and unsafe manufacturing of breast implants. For example, they found fault with Dow Corning Corporation, the leading manufacturer of implants, for withholding evidence from the public that these devices rupture and leak, or they pointed their fingers at the FDA for not taking a more active and aggressive approach toward regulating breast implants. Many other women I interviewed directed blame at their individual physicians—plastic surgeons who neglected to inform them of any possible health risks prior to their surgeries, and other doctors who continually minimized their concerns and dismissed their implant-related symptoms.

Most of my respondents, however, preferred not to single out specific individuals and agencies, but affixed blame on the entire health care system. These women understood their problems with breast implants within a larger political and economic context. For them, the root of their troubles lay in a health care system structured around the premise that making profits is of far greater importance than making people healthy. The women who had come to this realization were angry and outraged, feeling as if their physicians, as well as their government, had led them astray, down a precarious path of medical uncertainty. In order to explain why they were so misguided, many of these women had developed a "conspiracy theory," believing that the FDA, the medical community, and implant manufacturers had joined together to keep their implant-related troubles silent. Even though I argue that such a theory falls short of explaining the entire breast implant disaster,[1] the process of developing such an explanation, nevertheless, enabled many of the women I interviewed to transform their guilt and shame into anger and rage. These feelings, in turn, strengthened and reinforced women's convictions that their own negative experiences with implants were not simply isolated, personal troubles, but were a part of a much larger public issue.[2]

Anger and rage not only enabled women to locate the source of their troubles outside of themselves, but also to guide them out of their private, silent worlds and into the public arena. Indeed, hundreds of women who believe that they were misinformed about the risks associated with breast implants have become political about their experiences.[3] These women have joined together, forming national and local support groups and information networks for all implant recipients who are anxious and fearful about their futures. Many of these organizations not only provide support for individual women with breast implants and education about implant-related health problems, but they also encourage women to think about their personal troubles within a broader political context. Their newsletters illustrate ways in which they encourage women's politicization. For example, the headline of one California group's newsletter reads: "Speak Out on 'Tort Reform,'" urging women to write to their legislators opposing S.687, the Product Liability Fairness Act, a bill that, if passed, would impose severe restrictions on lawsuits against the manufacturers of injurious drugs and medical devices.[4] In the same issue, another headline reads: "March on LA," asking women to participate in a candlelight walk at the Los Angeles federal courthouse to protest the mishandling of the breast implant global settlement. Thus, women in support groups not only try to bring about a greater awareness of the problems inherent within our current health care system, but they also persistently find new ways to challenge the organization and structure of this system. In the process, they empower women to become better-informed consumers of health care.

Becoming political or adopting an activist stance toward one's illness is not a monocausal or linear process. In other words, there is no single variable that determines what leads some women to seek support and become political about their implant-related experiences and others to remain silent about these experiences. This point is reflected in the diversity of women who participate in support groups and have taken a political stance about their implant-related experiences. Abby, who leads her own support group, explained, "We have women from all walks of life—all different socioeconomic backgrounds, older women in their sixties and seventies who had breast cancer, young women who enlarged their breasts. Some are married, some single or divorced."

Despite the diversity among women who have sought support and validation for their experiences with breast implants, in this chapter I attempt to disentangle the factors that impel some women with breast implants to seek support and become political about their troubles, as well as the factors that lead other women to remain in the dark shadow of confusion and self-doubt. In so doing, I shed light on a decision that many women who have breast implants must confront: whether to place their faith in medical and scientific experts who base their knowledge on scientific "facts" about implant-related risk, or to have trust in their own knowledge about the source of their troubles. The distinction between these two approaches to knowledge resonates with the work of other social scientists who have explored and analyzed differences between knowledge based on medical and scientific "facts," and knowledge based on lay perceptions of health and illness. Elliot Mishler, for example, discusses this dichotomy in terms of two separate "voices" to explain how knowledge about health and illness is constructed differently for patients and their physicians.[5] Similarly, Phil Brown distinguishes between "lay and professional ways of knowing" about environmental health risk.[6] From the scientific and medical professions' viewpoint, risk can be determined only by controlled, epidemiological studies that are presumably value-neutral.[7] However, from the layperson's perspective, knowledge about risk can be acquired through personal life experiences. Such anecdotal evidence most often conflicts with the results of scientific studies that claim an "insignificant" relationship between exposure to toxins and disease.

My interview with Rebecca sheds light on differences between scientific and lay (or, what I term "intuitive") approaches to knowledge in the context of women's experiences with breast implants. Moreover, it reveals the tensions that arise as some women gradually become aware of the distinction between these two ways of knowing.

Wavering between Intuition and Scientific Evidence: An Interview with Rebecca

Rebecca is a middle-class white woman in her mid-forties. She is married, has two teen-age children, and is a part-time administrative assistant. Rebecca and her family live in a quiet, suburban neighborhood in New England. As we had arranged, I met Rebecca at her house in the late afternoon in the summer of 1994. She was the only one home since her children were off at summer camp and her husband was still at work. Since it was an unusually comfortable, cool day for the middle of July, Rebecca asked if I would mind if we sat outside. I happily acceded to her request, and after handing me a glass of lemonade and a fold-up chair, she led me out the door and onto the front lawn where we proceeded to set up for our interview. Since Rebecca's home was on top of a large hill, the setting provided an impressive view of the surrounding community, as well as a peaceful, quiet place for our meeting.

After unfolding our chairs and making ourselves comfortable, I began asking Rebecca questions about her life before and after her reconstructive surgery with breast implants in 1986. About a year prior to this surgery, Rebecca had a bilateral mastectomy following a diagnosis of breast cancer.[8] During the course of our interview, I learned that since Rebecca had received her implants, she had had numerous health problems, including pain in her chest and under her arms, sleep disturbances, difficulties with digestion, and irregular menstrual cycles. She also had been diagnosed with irritable bowel syndrome and fibromyalgia. Along with these autoimmune-related symptoms and illnesses, Rebecca also informed me that she has had a recurrence of cancer—about a year prior to our interview, Rebecca had undergone surgery for the removal of two malignant tumors—one in each of her ovaries.

Many of Rebecca's symptoms and diagnoses sounded nearly identical to those experienced by other women I had interviewed. Moreover, I had read about all of the types of problems she was experiencing in newsletters distributed by support groups and information networks for women with breast implants. Drawing from anecdotal evidence, these readings consistently make the claim that there is a strong correlation between silicone and autoimmune-related illness, contradicting findings from scientific studies that assert that this relationship is not significant. Rebecca, however, was not a member of a support group and, thus, had never seen a complete list of all the possible implant-related symptoms and illnesses. She had seen talk shows on television and read articles in newspapers that addressed the public and scientific controversy over breast implants, but for some reason, she was reluctant to view her problems in relation to other women's implant-related experiences and was unwilling to perceive her own implants as the cause of these troubles. Nevertheless, she had an analysis that differed from the dominant medical perspective. Rebecca's story is about a struggle that many of the other women I interviewed shared. This struggle is about what constitutes "accurate" knowledge, and the meaning of expertise. It also involves making an important and difficult decision: whether to rely on the prevailing belief that medicine and science are disciplines capable of discovering the only "truth" about disease causation, or to look beyond this assumption and develop a broader understanding of health and illness that includes life experiences and personal feelings about the source of one's troubles.

Rebecca hinted at the divergence between medical and scientific "facts," and her own feelings about the source of her troubles early on in our interview, after I had asked her to reflect on the way she felt following her reconstructive surgery. She responded:

> It seems that [problems started] after I had the surgery—not the mastectomy—after the mastectomy, within a month, I had full mobility and I felt absolutely wonderful. I probably even felt better than ever because I was maybe taking better care of myself. I just felt really well. After the reconstructive surgery, I never really felt that way again. I never felt free of discomfort or pain. And, I would ask all the doctors about [my implants]. Every doctor that I would see I would mention pain in my chest, pain under my arms, pain

in my ribs, difficulty sleeping because of pressure. And they would say "there is no evidence." So I would, you know, I would leave and I would ask every doctor that I saw. I figured that they would, you know, one out of four or five, if they were concerned would say something.

Comparing the way she felt after her mastectomy to the discomfort and pain she has experienced since her reconstructive surgery, Rebecca began to link her problems to her breast implants. She logically assumed that since she felt well after her mastectomy, and increasingly worse after her reconstructive surgery, her implants were to blame. This explanation made rational sense to her. However, at the same time, Rebecca could not completely trust her own suspicions about the source of her troubles, since every physician she had visited persistently told her that "there is no evidence" to support an association between her implants and her symptoms.

At this point in time, Rebecca had a great deal of respect for her doctors. She reported that the specialist who performed her mastectomy was written up in *Good Housekeeping*, and her plastic surgeon was an Ivy League graduate whose staff referred to him as "the miracle worker" and "an amazing artist." According to Rebecca, these characteristics were enough to assure her that the physicians she was choosing to visit were well qualified and knowledgeable. She had no reason to doubt their expertise and never thought about the possibility that they could provide her with misleading information. Thus, even though her intuition was at odds with her doctors' views that breast implants are "safe," she continued to rely on science and medicine for "accurate" information concerning her health.

This was not the only instance during our interview in which Rebecca revealed a disparity between her own beliefs about the cause of her health problems and her physicians' explanations for these troubles. During the years following her reconstructive surgery, Rebecca's pain progressively worsened and new problems had emerged, including fatigue, sleeplessness, and stomach irritability. In addition, Rebecca's menstrual cycles had become irregular. Putting all of these symptoms together, Rebecca thought for sure that she had a recurrence of cancer. Of course, she hoped that her suspicion was false, and she subsequently tried to come up with alternative explanations for her worsening health. For example, she said, "I thought [because of my irregular periods] that maybe I was premenopausal. This is what my doctors would say. When you have symptoms that are unexplainable and if you're in a certain age bracket, then they always seem to chalk it up to premenopause." At this point during our interview, Rebecca began to hint at her underlying apprehension about physicians' expertise. Viewing her troubles in the larger context of other women's experiences with doctors who wrongly attribute their symptoms to their reproductive functioning,[9] she began to question "medical" explanations for disease causation. Furthermore, Rebecca felt that premenopause seemed like an illogical label for her own problem since the distance between her periods was becoming shorter, not growing further apart. Again, despite the logic behind her own suspicions, and her misgivings about "premenopause" as an accurate diagnosis, she favored this "medical" explanation, hoping to find a reason for the decline in her health.

Although Rebecca felt uneasy that her doctor was attributing her symptoms to early menopause, she was reassured when he told her that, in addition to checking her hormonal levels for this condition, he would also perform an endometrial biopsy and an ultrasound to rule out cancer. All of the results of these tests were "normal." In other words, according to the medical evidence, Rebecca was not experiencing early menopause, nor did she have cancer. Despite this good news, a voice inside of Rebecca kept tugging away at her, telling her that something was still terribly wrong. If everything was "fine," why was she continuing to experience such strange symptoms? She expressed these concerns to her gynecologist, who replied that there was nothing else he could do and recommended that she visit another specialist—perhaps her symptoms were not the result of a reproductive malfunction, but were caused by a problem elsewhere in her body.

Rebecca took her gynecologist's advice and decided to visit a gastroenterologist. She was quite pleased with the doctor he had recommended because, out of all the physicians she had seen, the gastroenterologist was the only one who "listened to everything I said. And, based on what I said, conducted all of the appropriate tests." Again, Rebecca's comment illustrates a subtle shift in the meaning she attributed to medical "expertise." Just as she had begun to question the competence of physicians who attribute women's troubles to reproductive processes, at this point during our interview she also began to question the overall characteristics of a good doctor. She had once believed that the most qualified doctors were those who had prestigious educational backgrounds ("Ivy League" graduates), or had been written up in popular magazines. Now, however, a more important characteristic of a medical expert is someone who is an attentive listener and who is willing to collaborate with a patient to come up with a plausible diagnosis.

After a series of examinations and tests, Rebecca's gastroenterologist diagnosed her with irritable bowel syndrome. For a short time, Rebecca accepted this diagnosis and focused on ways to change her lifestyle in order to make herself more comfortable with this condition: She changed her diet and began exercising daily. Despite these efforts, Rebecca's stomach problems did not improve. In addition, her periods were still irregular and she continued to experience pains in her chest, general achiness, and chronic fatigue. Once again, Rebecca began to suspect that her symptoms were indicative of a more serious illness than what her doctors were leading her to believe. In the back of her mind, she still thought that she had some form of cancer.

Concerned and frightened, Rebecca returned to her gynecologist, who agreed to perform a laparoscopy to see if he could find anything unusual in her uterus or ovaries. Again, all of her tests came back "normal." Given these results, the gynecologist explained to Rebecca that there was nothing wrong with her. He performed a dilation and curettage (D and C) to regulate her periods, and sent her on her way. Rebecca's health improved somewhat after this visit—her periods seemed to return to normal, and her strict, fiber-rich diet finally seemed to control her irritable bowel condition. Moreover, she felt a great sense of relief knowing that she "had done everything that [she] had needed to" to rule out her suspicion about cancer. Even though she continued to experience sleeplessness and pain in her abdomen, she went about her daily life without worrying about these symptoms. When Rebecca went back to her gynecologist the following year for an annual checkup, he reassured her again that "everything looked fine."

A few months later, a couple of nights before Rebecca was to make her trip into the city for her six-month breast exam, she was awakened in the middle of the night, feeling a large mass in her abdomen. She tried not to become alarmed, convincing herself that her hand was simply pressing against her full bladder. Knowing that she had an appointment at her medical center in just a few days also set her at ease. She would mention the mass to her doctors and, in the meantime, would not worry.

Rebecca normally took the train into town and then walked from the station to her appointment. The distance on foot was "quite a hike," but Rebecca said that she had always liked to walk and never had any problems—until this particular day. After taking just a few strides away from the station, she doubled over with abdominal pain and felt nauseous and dizzy. Despite her condition, Rebecca somehow managed to get herself to her appointment at the medical center. Upon her arrival, she told her doctors about her frightening experience and also expressed to them her concern about the mass in her abdomen. Even though she was certain that something was seriously wrong with her, to her surprise, her physicians did not seem terribly concerned:

> My doctor examined me and didn't notice anything. They didn't give me a pelvic exam, they just gave me the usual: Check the breasts, check my heart, check my lungs. . . . One doctor felt my abdomen but didn't seem concerned about the discomfort I had and seemed to disregard the whole episode of me not being able to walk there and having pain in my "lower right quadrant" (that is what they call it). I explained to them all of the tests I had in prior years, and they just said to me, "Well, you passed your breast exam and you don't have to come back for another year." I said to my regular doctor, "Well, what about all these symptoms, you know—the stomach, irritable bowel syndrome, the pain—I can't walk!?" And he said, "Well, you might want to get in touch with an internist."

The anger resonated in Rebecca's voice as she repeated this physician's response to her concerns: "You *might* want to consider getting in touch with an internist." She explained, "I didn't like hearing those words at all."

Out of all of the doctors Rebecca had visited, she had felt most comfortable with her gastroenterologist: "I just felt that if anybody is going to take my concerns seriously and do anything or feel anything or perform the right tests and not just say that I'm premenopausal or that I'm hysterical or, whatever—he'll be the one." This doctor agreed to see Rebecca right away and, upon examining her, immediately felt the mass in her abdomen. The next day, Rebecca went to the hospital for further tests, and an ultrasound alone revealed large masses in each of her ovaries. That day, Rebecca's intuition was validated. Indeed, she did have a recurrence of cancer. Shortly after her diagnosis, she had a complete hysterectomy and began chemotherapy. Rebecca had finished this therapy a few months prior to our interview and reported that her prognosis is good. However, she still was troubled. None of the symptoms she experienced prior to the onset of her cancer—the sleeplessness, aching joints, and stomach irritability—had gone away, and, in fact, they had worsened.

The oncologist who had treated Rebecca's ovarian cancer had no explanation for her continuing health problems. Frustrated and "displeased with the general medical scenario," Rebecca turned to a holistic health center where an allergist conducted a series of blood tests that indicated that she had an autoimmune-related illness called fibromyalgia. This doctor also explained to Rebecca that he had heard that many women with breast implants had been diagnosed with this condition. Rebecca had difficulty absorbing this information, explaining to me, "I really just didn't want to hear that my implants were the cause of all of my problems. I don't want to have more surgery, I don't want to have to go back to scratch—you know, back to square one." In other words, Rebecca not only feared the thought of surgery to remove her implants but, even more so, she dreaded the idea of returning to a body without breasts.

However, Rebecca was skeptical of her allergist's "holistic" practices. And, even though she felt at ease with him and accepted his diagnosis of fibromyalgia, she was unwilling to place her faith in his belief that her implants were causing her troubles. Part of this unwillingness stemmed from the scientific and medical community's reluctance to make claims about a relationship between implants and disease: "The doctors in the medical profession who really believe in scientific tests and the scientific method saying that the majority of women do not have problems with implants—this is what I prefer to believe."

Despite her fears about implant removal and doubts about holistic healers, throughout our interview Rebecca increasingly revealed her suspicion that her implants had some connection with her worsening health. For instance, she alluded to this belief after telling me that, while in her attic, she had come across the breast prosthesis that she had worn following her mastectomy and before her reconstructive surgery. The device was made of silicone and had completely deteriorated, oozing a gooey, sticky gel all over the place. Upon seeing this, Rebecca immediately thought to herself, "My God, this is what is inside of me?!" Later on in our interview, she further explained, "In the back of my mind, I really suspect that—I mean, so far, my intuition has been right about everything else. I mean, I knew I had ovarian cancer long before any of these doctors did. And, if I am honest with myself, in the back of my mind, I suspect that the implants are responsible for at least some of the symptoms I am having, because they have all started after the implants and they haven't gotten better. They have gotten worse—even with the elimination of cancer." Nevertheless, Rebecca's damaged silicone prosthesis and her suspicions about her breast implants were not enough to completely convince her of an association between these devices and her worsening symptoms: "I guess I am waiting for either things to get worse or for the medical science group to come out and finally say—I guess, still, they are the ones that I really trust."

During the course of our interview, Rebecca's intuition about the source of her problems was continually at odds with the scientific and medical evidence concerning these troubles. For instance, the tests her doctors performed on her to rule out cancer came back "normal"; and yet, she continued to suspect that something was still terribly wrong with her. In a sense, Rebecca considered herself "lucky" since she had been reading about cancer and was quite "tuned in" to her body. She explained, "I was watchful and just didn't let things rest. I went to the doctors and kept pushing and pushing." In this case, Rebecca's intuition about the source of her worsening health prevailed over the scientific and medical evidence. Her persistent belief that she had cancer drove her to become actively involved in her own health care decisions, leading her, finally, to the diagnosis she had been waiting to hear. After an ultrasound, her doctor confirmed her long-standing suspicion that she did, in fact, have cancer.

Rebecca's experiences with most of her doctors (aside from the gastroenterologist) prior to her cancer diagnosis led her to increasingly doubt medical "facts" and "expertise." This disillusionment stemmed from her doctors' persistent unwillingness or inability to listen to, or consider, her own thoughts about the reasons for her worsening health. In effect, medical "experts," or those who were supposed to be knowledgeable about health, illness, and disease causation, continually failed to respond to her health problems and concerns in a way that made sense to her.

Rebecca's dissatisfaction with her physicians led her to seek an alternative approach to health care—she went to the holistic health center for help. At the center, the allergist explained to her that the silicone from her implants may have triggered an immune reaction in her body that would account for her worsening symptoms. Since Rebecca's health did not improve after the treatment for her ovarian cancer, she, too, began to suspect that her implants were to blame. Nevertheless, she was not completely convinced since, first, her allergist was not a real medical doctor, but had "some kind of doctoral degree in an obscure field of science" and, second, the scientific evidence suggests that there is no significant relationship between implants and disease. Rebecca's fears about implant removal—the prospect of another surgery and the thought of replacing her breasts, once again, with a concave chest wall—also contributed to her reliance on scientific evidence. Even though her inner voice had been accurate before (when it told her that she had cancer), she now was hesitant to let this same voice prevail over scientific and medical reasoning and logic. Rather than considering herself an expert on the source of her health problems, Rebecca wavered between her intuition and the scientific evidence regarding breast implants. Toward the end of our interview, she explained, "I am still rolling the dice and waiting for all the facts to come in. . . . I'm waiting to see what happens and who ends up being closest to the truth."

Implicit in Rebecca's decision to wait for all the medical and scientific "facts" to "come in," is the idea that there is only one underlying "truth" about breast implants and disease causation, and that the only ones capable of discovering this truth are medical and scientific experts. This belief is infused with predominating cultural assumptions about medicine and science. In Western society, knowledge based on medical and scientific evidence is presumed to be legitimate, accurate, and rational. However, knowledge based on intuition is relegated to the realm of conjecture and speculation—only verifiable when brought into the scientific arena where the appropriate tests can be applied.[10] As I have demonstrated in earlier chapters, these assumptions are misleading since medical and scientific knowledge about implanted-related risks has always been uncertain, ambiguous, and vague.

In one sense, Rebecca's interview sheds light on a dichotomy between knowledge based on scientific or medical "facts" and knowledge based on feelings and life experiences. However, her experience also illuminates how a "dichotomy" between two different approaches to knowledge is unable to capture the complex process through which individuals make sense of different types of evidence. Rebecca *wavers* between the scientific and personal evidence, without choosing which type of knowledge most accurately defines her own situation. A dichotomy also ignores how an individual's approach to knowledge can change over time. When Rebecca's health began to deteriorate, her intuition about ovarian cancer prevailed over the results of medical tests indicating that nothing was wrong with her. However, when her health continued to deteriorate after completing her cancer treatments, the medical and scientific evidence prevailed over her own suspicions about her worsening symptoms. In other words, because scientific studies do not confirm a relationship between implants and disease, Rebecca assumed that her suspicions about implants and her deteriorating health must be inaccurate.

Variations among Individual Approaches to Knowledge: Resisting Politicization

Susan Bell's analysis of her interview with a woman who had a miscarriage as a consequence of her prenatal exposure to diethylstilbestrol (DES) similarly shows how personal beliefs about knowledge and expertise can change over time.[11] Bell interprets three stories that emerged during the course of her interaction with a woman she calls Sarah in order to illustrate the process of "becoming a political woman." For Sarah, this process involved a gradual shift in her focus away from medical explanations, which attributed her miscarriage to a bodily defect, toward a greater reliance on her own beliefs about the source of her troubles.

Sarah's doctor attributed her miscarriage not only to her exposure to DES, but also to her "incompetent" cervix. Sarah initially accepted this explanation and, subsequently, linked her inability to carry a pregnancy to term to her identity as a DES daughter, as well as a malfunction within her own body. Over time, however, she began to connect her exposure to DES to further problems. For instance, she gradually came to realize that her loss could have been prevented—her doctor should not have prescribed DES to her mother and, more important, her doctor "should have known that she was at risk of a miscarriage."[12] Sarah began to recognize that "medical logic is fallible" and that it "is not the only voice that [could] explain her situation."[13] Sarah's willingness to question medical knowledge allowed her to see that her troubles were not simply isolated and private, but shared by other women exposed to DES. Making this connection led Sarah to join DES Action, a national organization that not only collects and distributes information about DES, but also "attempts to change laws and regulations regarding medical services for these women."[14] Sarah had become "a political woman."

Sarah's story is similar to Rebecca's in many ways. First, each woman had been exposed to a substance that has potential iatrogenic, or treatment-induced, health effects. Sarah's mother had taken DES during her pregnancy with Sarah, and Rebecca had received breast implants made of silicone. Second, these women both experienced symptoms or conditions that were possibly linked to their exposure to these substances. Sarah had a miscarriage that may be attributed to her prenatal exposure to DES, and Rebecca experienced a number of autoimmune symptoms potentially related to her silicone breast implants. Finally, both women talked about their increasing dissatisfaction with medicine, as their physicians continually failed to come up with explanations for their troubles that made sense to them.

In Sarah's case, her gradual disappointment with her doctors coincided with her ability to shift blame away from her own body (or, her "incompetent" cervix) and direct it at medicine for "exposing her to DES and failing to warn her of reproductive risks associated with this exposure."[15] Sarah had come to recognize the limitations of medical and scientific knowledge, allowing her to see that her own DES-related health problems were not merely personal and private troubles but were shared by other women exposed to the drug. Her involvement with DES Action continually validated her belief that her individual experiences with DES were a part of a much larger social and political issue.

Rebecca, too, had increasingly become disappointed with medicine. She found that most of her doctors were not taking her fears and concerns about cancer seriously, nor were they providing her with a plausible reason for her wide range of symptoms. In this case, Rebecca was willing to accept the limitations of medical and scientific knowledge and, relying on her intuition, visited her doctors until they finally diagnosed her with ovarian cancer. However, Rebecca was reluctant to accept these same limitations when it came to questions regarding breast implants. In this case, she continually placed her trust in the scientific evidence and was unable to connect her personal feelings and experiences with those of other implant recipients. Thus, while Rebecca and Sarah's narratives are similar, they also are very different. Rebecca had not become political about her experiences with implants because, unlike Sarah, she resisted trying to make sense of her private troubles within a larger social and political context. For instance, when I asked Rebecca if she had tried to contact other women with breast implants, she replied, "No, I really don't want to believe there is a problem with them. And, I don't want to start thinking that every ache and pain I have is a result of the implants." Similarly, she explained that the reason she had not attempted to find a support group was that "I didn't want to be persuaded. . . . I didn't want to put myself in a position where I would start hearing other women's problems and start thinking I had the same problems."

Other women I interviewed felt similarly about connecting with other women with breast implants. For instance, like Rebecca, Leslie told me that she suspected that her implants could be causing her troubles, but was reluctant to join a support group. This reluctance may have been linked to her ambivalence toward the scientific evidence regarding breast implants: "The jury appears to be still out. Maybe this is my denial but, then again, my belief [about implants] isn't being proven right now." Without the scientific "proof" that breast implants are dangerous, Rebecca, Leslie, and other women I spoke with could not trust their own intuitions about implants. One explanation for this resistance may relate to women's fear of implant removal. For instance, Eve commented, "Removal is a really big issue. I think some woman, myself included, sit and weigh out whether or not breast implants are really life-threatening and is it really worth getting disfigured over." [16] Similarly, Rebecca explained that since she had already lost her breasts due to cancer once, she certainly did not want to lose them again. Sarah, on the other hand, did not have to pay this kind of penalty for breaking away from the predominating voice of medicine and trusting her own knowledge about DES. In effect, while Sarah could understand her private troubles within a broader social and political context, Rebecca and many other women I interviewed could not.

Troubles with Implants Are "Not My Problem"

Some of the women I interviewed resisted connecting their experiences with those of other implant recipients simply because they had no reason to doubt the scientific evidence suggesting that implants are safe. Indeed, not every woman with implants has experienced symptoms they believe to be implant-related. For example, in my sample of forty, six women reported that they were in good health and had not exhibited any symptoms they thought were related to their implants. [17] Four of these women could not see how they could possibly identify with the women who claimed to be having implant-related troubles. [18] Maureen, for example, referred to these women as "the ones who are jumping on the bandwagon." Carmen also never considered contacting other women with breast implants since she had saline implants and believed that the women who were experiencing problems were only those who had the implants made out of silicone.

Mary, who had received two breast implants after a bilateral mastectomy at the age of sixty-four in 1986, also could not see how her life experiences were similar to those of other women with implants. After reading an article in her local newspaper about the possible health effects of migrating silicone, she did become "a little concerned" and decided to attend a local support group meeting for women with breast implants. However, she explained:

> Some of the women [in the group] were these young girls who had implants for cosmetic reasons and they were having a lot of problems. There was one woman who went to a doctor out in Texas and, she has something serious. I don't know that it could be blamed on the implants. And, it was so sad to me because they would cry sometimes when they would be telling me their stories. And, I thought, I don't need this. There wasn't much I could do to help them. So, if I couldn't help anybody, then I didn't see any point in going and getting depressed over somebody else's problems. So, I stopped going.

Even though Mary had experienced problems with her own implants (ruptures, requiring a total of three replacement surgeries, and capsular contracture), she could not identify with the women in the support group since most of them were much younger than herself; they had had implants for "cosmetic" reasons rather than reconstructive purposes and were reporting symptoms that she herself had never experienced. Detaching herself from the group, Mary was able to continue denying any possible relationship between silicone and autoimmune illness (i.e., the woman who went to Texas had a serious health problem, but her implants were not necessarily to blame).

Maureen, Carmen, and Mary had not experienced any implant-related autoimmune symptoms, nor had they expressed concern about developing future health problems related to their breast implants; therefore, they saw no reason to be angry with their physicians or skeptical of the scientific evidence suggesting that implants are safe. In their minds, their perceived positive experiences with breast implants gave credence to this evidence and, thus, supported the legitimacy of medical and scientific knowledge.

However, most of the women I interviewed did not report such good outcomes following their plastic surgeries. Many talked not only about ruptured, failed implants, but also about a slow progression of strange symptoms. Thirty-four of the women I interviewed believed that these symptoms were associated with their implants. Even some of these women resisted connecting their symptoms and diseases to similar troubles experienced by other implant recipients. For instance, Beth told me that she had been experiencing sleeplessness, chronic infections, digestive problems, and joint pain for a number of years. Although she suspected that these symptoms were related to the implants she had received in 1981, she was reluctant to talk to women who were possibly sharing similar types of troubles: "I don't want to put myself in a support group where everybody is unhealthy. . . . I can't take on *anybody else's* [emphasis added] problems."

Although Beth's comment suggests that she did not join a group because she did not want to be burdened with other women's problems, it also sheds light on her denial about her own troubles. Beth, too, was "unhealthy," experiencing numerous autoimmune-related symptoms; nevertheless, she found comfort and reassurance in perceiving a distinction between her own symptoms and those of other women who had implants. Like other women I spoke with, Beth explained how her denial was exacerbated by her doctors' conviction that her symptoms were not implant-related. Not sure about whether to place her faith in these medical "experts," or to listen to her own inner voice, she commented, "Does the fact that someone has an M.D. behind their name make them smarter than me? I struggle with this on an internal level because I have been sick and have not been able to finish college. So, I feel stupid and that maybe I should believe these doctors. But then, there is this little voice inside that is saying something else. Should I blindly believe my doctors, or should I work on this little voice?"

The Consequences of Acknowledging a Problem

Women's resistance to probing into the roots of their troubles may be related to potential consequences involved in acknowledging a link between their worsening health and their implants. For instance, many women believed that if they admitted that their troubles were linked to their implants, they would inevitably have to confront the prospect of having these devices removed. This was the case for Georgine.

Georgine is a thirty-two-year-old model who is married and has a five-year-old daughter. She received her breast implants in 1990, hoping this would advance her career. Shortly after her surgery, she and her husband had decided to have another child; however, Georgine had difficulties becoming pregnant. When she finally did conceive, she had a miscarriage six weeks into her pregnancy. Georgine told me that she was certain that her implants were somehow associated with her fertility problems: "I really feel that my problems are due to the implants and my autoimmune response and things like that. I can't say it is for sure—but I would bet. And I have been trying to get pregnant ever since and it has been two or three years and—even with infertility drugs, I haven't been successful." However, she also explained to me that she was not always so willing to make this connection between her implants and her personal troubles.

About a year after Georgine had received her implants, she began hearing about possible dangers related to the devices on talk shows and news reports and became increasingly concerned. One of the talk shows had mentioned a national network for women with breast implants. Georgine jotted down the address and decided to write to the group for information. The group sent her newsletters that were filled with women's accounts of their ruptured, defective implants, and lists of their debilitating autoimmune symptoms and diseases. Georgine was shocked as she read this information and became terribly upset. She could not bear to face the possibility that she herself might someday experience the same types of troubles that these women were reporting. Moreover, she thought the consequences of acknowledging a potential link between silicone and disease were intolerable—admitting this link meant confronting the prospect of implant removal. Even though Georgine "knew in the back of [her] mind that [she] would have to face this situation," for the time being, she preferred to disregard the information in the newsletters. She explained, "I didn't want to get rid of my breasts." Thus, rather than identifying with the women who were experiencing numerous implant-related troubles, Georgine chose to see herself as "different" from them. Although the newsletters from the information network continued to appear in the mail, she simply stuffed them away and out of sight in a kitchen drawer, thinking that the whole implant controversy would eventually "blow over."

Hillary was a nurse who used to work in a plastic surgeon's office. After learning that she had had her own breast implants removed, I asked her if she could provide me with some insight into why other women, who suspected that their implants were causing them health problems, might decide against this surgery.[19] She explained, "I think there are two things. First, there is the fear associated with the body image change and, also, another surgery. The second thing is that plastic surgeons keep telling women not to get them out—that there is 'no problem.'" Although Hillary gave me two separate explanations, they really are interrelated: The dreadful thought of returning to a flat-chested body compels women to cling to their doctors' assertions that there is "no problem" with breast implants. Thus, rather than probing into the roots of their troubles, many women preferred to accept the prevailing assumption that medical knowledge is more legitimate than their own intuitive feelings about the source of their troubles.

Rose offers another possible reason why women may deny a link between their worsening health and their implants. Rose was an active member of a support group for women with breast implants and, through a friend, had met a woman whose entire family was unaware that she had implants. Even though Rose urged this woman to come to a group meeting, the women replied: "If I go, I may see somebody I know. And nobody knows." Rose continued, saying, "This poor woman had all of these autoimmune disorders already diagnosed by doctors who didn't even know that she has implants." Thus, some women may resist acknowledging any problems with their implants because they are afraid of being "found out." Hillary's comment supports this explanation: "Having breast implants is a pretty personal issue. It is not something you discuss with someone on the street, you know, because people will make assumptions about you. In fact, one doctor told me, 'I have never known a woman with breast implants that isn't crazy.' I guess he didn't know that I had breast implants."

Class and Ethnic Barriers to Finding Support[20]

Barbara had a different reason for not seeking support or validation for her troubles with breast implants. She was born and raised in South America and had immigrated to the United States with her brother when they were young adults. When I visited Barbara in 1994, she and her brother were living together in a tiny, cluttered, one-bedroom apartment in a working-class neighborhood on the outskirts of a large city. Barbara had a part-time job as a nurse and was supporting her brother, who was currently unemployed. Barbara was experiencing many implant-related problems. However, her busy work schedule, along with her poor economic situation, prevented her from dwelling on the extent of her pain and discomfort.

Moreover, Barbara admitted that "there is economic pressures all over the world" but explained that coping with these pressures in

America was particularly difficult: "The social environment in this country is very bad. There is no sense of community where you can make friends and socialize. Back where I am from, people are more open and giving. If we need anything, people will do things without expecting you to do another favor." Already feeling detached from American culture, Barbara resigned herself to silence and isolation when she began experiencing troubles with her implants. These problems arose shortly after she received her implants in 1972. One of the devices had ruptured, and silicone had migrated into her surrounding breast tissue. Barbara had the implant replaced but, since this surgery, has been experiencing severe pains in her chest and right arm, which frequently impedes her ability to work. Although she had read a few articles about the possible dangers of silicone implants in the early 1990s, and suspected that her own implants were causing her pain, she had more important things to worry about than her health: "I am just trying to get by. I cope with my day even when I am uncomfortable and in a lot of pain. I put this pain in the closet, close the closet, and go about my life trying to make the best of my day. And then, when I come back at night I think about opening the closet. But, no—I stopped reading about breast implants." Similarly, when I asked Barbara if she had tried to talk to other women who had breast implants, she said, "This implant issue is a very hard thing to face every day, from my personal experience. As I said, I put it in the closet and go on with other problems in my life that need to be dealt with. Whether this is good or bad, I don't know. But this is what I am doing. And, I don't know or care what other women are doing." In other words, Barbara was more concerned about how she and her brother were going to make it through each day, given their poor financial situation, than with how she was going to cope with her problems with implants. Her reason for not seeking support or validation from other implant recipients was not necessarily related to her unwillingness to identify with the troubles experienced by these women, but was linked more to her inability to place her daily life struggles as a working-class woman aside so that she could focus on her own health.[21]

The Persistent Search for Answers

While many of the women I interviewed resisted finding support for their suspicions about breast implants, others were so convinced that their health problems were implant-related that they found themselves on a persistent search for validation of this belief. These women were no longer silent about their fears and concerns and were ready to accept the consequences of acknowledging a link between their implants and their worsening health—even if this meant returning to their old, flat-chested bodies. However, most women who were willing to trust their intuition and accept the limitations of scientific studies found themselves facing bleak moments of despair and self-doubt, as they trudged onward in their search, hoping to find someone who would understand the extent of their fears, pains, and frustrations.

Some women eventually found a compassionate listener. For example, before Gloria started her own support group for women with breast implants, she had doubted her suspicions about her implants because her plastic surgeon continually dismissed her troubles, telling her they were all "in her head." He further told Gloria that she needed to see a psychiatrist. Filled with self-doubt and confusion, Gloria took his advice: "I needed somebody to talk to. I didn't know what was happening." Ironically, the psychiatrist took Gloria's symptoms and concerns quite seriously. He said that he did not believe that she was imagining her symptoms and encouraged her to conduct her own research on breast implants. Moreover, he told her that he, too, would search for some answers that might provide an explanation for the way she had been feeling. Together, Gloria and her psychiatrist came up with enough literature on breast implants to validate Gloria's long-standing belief that the silicone from these devices was causing her troubles.

Leslie also doubted her intuition about breast implants until she found a similar kind of support from an attorney handling breast implant litigation. She thought that the joint pain and chronic sore throats she had been experiencing could be related to the implants she had received in 1986, but since all of her doctors told her she was "fine" and no medical test confirmed a problem, she decided not to be concerned. Nevertheless, she had read a newspaper article about an attorney who was handling breast implant litigation, and decided to call simply to get more information. She made an appointment but, after her visit, decided not to pursue the implant issue any further, telling herself that her symptoms were not serious. However, the lawyer continued to send Leslie information about the possible long-term health effects of breast implants and asked Leslie if she could pay her a visit: "She met me here at my house and we went through everything. She had me getting my medical records and I started putting things together and making my own chart and looking at everything that I could get a hold of. And, I just felt at the end of that meeting, there was really no denying that I really had this set pattern of things that had happened only after receiving the implants." When I met Leslie in 1994, she was not entirely ready to face the consequences of acknowledging a link between her implants and her symptoms; however, knowing that she had her lawyer to turn to for support and understanding made her feel at ease. Similarly, Eve commented: "My attorney feels as strongly as I do that my problems are related and, it is nice to have somebody to support me like that."

Unfortunately, many of the women I interviewed never found this kind of support through a caring and attentive listener. Joyce, for example, explained, "For two years now, I had been trying to prove that something was wrong with my implants and everybody was telling me it is all in my head, even though I knew that something was wrong." Nevertheless, Joyce eventually did find validation. In her case, an X ray of her ruptured implant confirmed her belief about the relationship between her implants and her poor health. Moreover, it provided her with the medical proof necessary to convince her physicians, who had continually dismissed her troubles, that she was not "going crazy": "I remember getting the result of the MRI [magnetic resonance imaging] back. I was as happy as I was the day my children were born. My mind was given back to me. You know, finally, somebody was going to take me seriously. And, I can remember celebrating in glory over there on the couch and, then, all of a sudden realizing, that this is sick: I am actually happy over the fact that my implant is ruptured? You know, what is wrong with this picture? This is really pathetic. But, you know, my dignity was back, my self respect. And, now I know I wasn't crazy." Patty had a similar reaction after she learned about her rupture: "It wasn't until I actually had a rupture when I could say, 'Nobody is going to tell me I am crazy now.'"

And, Brenda, who was diagnosed with an implant-related autoimmune disease, explained, "The day that I found out that I actually had something—there is not too many women who could tell you that they were happy they have a disease. But, I was very happy. I was very happy." Continually doubting their suspicions about implants and unable to find support for their troubles, these women, ironically, were delighted when they finally had a name to give their troubles.

The Role of Support Groups

In their efforts to find validation for their troubles, many of the women I interviewed also attempted to find support and understanding through other women who shared similar concerns, fears, and health problems as their own. In fact, twenty out of the forty women I interviewed had either joined or started their own support group for women with breast implants. Karen referred to the members of her support group as her "extended family," further stating: "My sisters through the breast implant support network have been the ones who really understand. . . . These are the women who can identify with my rage, my fear and pain." Similarly, Gloria, who had started her own support group, explained: "The women who joined my group made me realize that I was not alone. I really felt that I had a common bond with somebody who understood how I was feeling. And, not only that, they made me feel good that I was starting to find information that was also helpful to others and, in turn, as they were getting things done and dealing with their own business with silicone problems, they were able to seek more information. We were helping each other now. We became a network." These women's willingness to relate their own life situations to the experiences of other implant recipients enabled them to transform their feelings of self-doubt and fear into anger and rage. For instance, at one support group meeting that Paula had attended, she became "very indignant that the [implant] manufacturers had acted in such a way. You know, I was starting to learn about the real corporate crime that I felt had been committed. I started to learn that it wasn't just me and one pair of silicone implants." Moreover, their ability to identify with other women who were in circumstances similar to their own allowed them to understand the limits of medical and scientific knowledge and have faith in their own suspicions about the source of their troubles. For example, only after Frances had connected with a support group did she realize that medical tests and her physicians, who continually told her that nothing was wrong with her, could be fallible: "Every doctor I go to—they don't know what is wrong with me. Everything shows up negative. So, then I called this lady from the support group and, sure enough, everything I said about my health—she could verify it."

Support groups not only validate women's experiences, enabling them to trust their own intuitive ways of knowing about health and illness, but in so doing, they also transform women's identities. Eleanor, for instance, had so many health problems after receiving her implants that she began to consider herself an ill-tempered complainer. She was so unhappy with herself that she simply wanted "to take some pills and be left alone." However, she changed her mind when a friend of hers brought her to a support group: "At the meeting I started hearing the word 'empowerment.' People were telling me what a nice person I am—nice things. I was hearing nice things. I was hearing women—educated women—saying very nice things about me."

Joining support groups, finding an interested and caring listener, or receiving a positive result on a medical test that confirmed a ruptured implant or an autoimmune illness were the factors that led many of the women I interviewed to believe that their troubles were not imaginary, but related to their breast implants. Once these women made this connection, they could break away from the dominant medical and scientific perspective that perpetuated the belief that their problems were all in their heads, not in their bodies. They no longer relied on medical and scientific explanations for answers about the risks associated with breast implants, but trusted their own intuition about health, illness, and disease causation.

Other women I interviewed, however, were unable to break away from the prevailing voice of medical science. Some readily accepted the scientific evidence that suggests that implants and disease are not significantly related because they had more urgent needs in their lives to attend to than their health. For instance, Barbara was more concerned about how she and her brother were going to survive on her limited income than she was about acknowledging the possibility that her implants were connected to her worsening symptoms. Women who were unable to accept the consequences of implant removal also resisted following their own instincts about the source of their troubles. Afraid of not only returning to a flat or concave chest wall, but also the possibility of permanent scarring and disfigurement, these women preferred to rely on the scientific "facts" about implant-related risk, while denying the existence of their own health problems. Even though some of these women suspected that the symptoms they were experiencing were related to their breast implants, they chose not to listen to their own inner voices.

8

Transforming Identities
Experiences of Empowerment

K athy Davis's research on women's experiences with cosmetic surgery[1] included follow-up interviews with twelve women one year after they had received breast implants. All of these women reported experiencing some pain and discomfort related to their surgeries, ranging from loss of nipple sensation to extreme hardening of the breasts and encapsulation. Some of these women had also developed infections leading to multiple operations on their chests and permanent scarring. Despite these troubles, Davis discovered that most of her respondents were "willing to accept their disappointing results and take on more than their share of the responsibility [for them]."[2] For instance, after Caroline received her implants, an abscess developed in her right breast, causing her implant to break through her incisions. She had to undergo three additional surgeries to correct for the problem, leaving massive scars across her chest. Nevertheless, Davis explains that Caroline remained "very proud that she didn't give up" and "was glad to have had the surgery."[3] She did not regret her decision to have undergone cosmetic surgery, nor did she perceive herself as a "hapless victim of fate." Rather, she portrayed herself as an "agent in interaction with her circumstances."[4]

During the course of Davis's research, she met only one woman, Irene, who was certain that she would not have

chosen to have implants if she had been aware of the possible consequences of this surgery. Unlike the other women in Davis's sample who,
at the time they were interviewed, had had their implants for only a
year, Irene had had her surgery "more than fifteen years ago."[5] In her
case, breast augmentation resulted in constant infections, encapsulation, a total of fifteen repeated surgeries on her chest, and permanent
disfigurement. Moreover, she had developed disabling rheumatic
symptoms: chronic fatigue, difficulty walking, and constant pain. Most
of the women I interviewed had also had many years of experience with
breast implants and reported similar types of debilitating symptoms and
complications. In earlier chapters, I described how many of these
women felt betrayed by medical experts who dismissed and minimized
their implant-related troubles and concerns. Davis reports that Irene
felt similarly. She, too, felt victimized by her physicians, who failed to
take her symptoms seriously, treating her as if she was "just some hysterical complainer."[6] Irene and the majority of women I interviewed
wished they had never placed their trust in their doctors and regretted
having unwittingly traded their health for their appearance.

At first glance, Irene's case seems to contradict Davis's argument
that, for some women "cosmetic surgery may be a resource for empowerment"[7] or, the best choice taken to alleviate their own personal suffering. Davis herself states that Irene "personifies the nightmare of
having an operation which leaves one in far worse shape than before
surgery."[8] However, Davis also presents a positive dimension to Irene's
ordeal. Instead of giving up when her doctors dismissed her problems,
Irene decided "to take [her] place at the helm," and conducted her own
investigation of the risks associated with breast implants. The more
she read about the possible health effects of silicone, the manufacturer
cover-ups, and the contradictory scientific findings, the more infuriated
and frightened she became. Even though she was angry, Irene increasingly became aware of her own ability to educate herself about the complicated effects of silicone and the history of breast implants. She took
pride in these accomplishments and began educating other implant recipients about the possible dangers of the devices. According to Davis,
Irene's pain and suffering, ironically, had made her a stronger person:
"Paradoxically, cosmetic surgery disrupted her life, but in so doing
also provided an opportunity for her to renegotiate her identity; after
it her life took a turn for the better. For Irene, cosmetic surgery has

been profoundly disempowering and a road to empowerment at the same time."[9]

Many of the women I interviewed who had experienced numerous implant-related health problems and complications talked about similar identity transformations. For instance, Brenda, who had developed debilitating rheumatic symptoms after receiving implants, reflected: "I have learned an awful lot [since receiving implants]. I have learned about myself, and I have got a wealth of knowledge I would have never had before. [My experiences with implants] have made me perhaps a more interesting person, a much more relaxed person and, maybe my new life to come will not be—will be much easier because I have gone through all of this." And, Tracy, who had her implants removed because she was terribly concerned about the possibility of developing implant-related diseases explained, "My experience with implants has taught me an awful lot. It has changed me in many ways. It has made me feistier and not afraid of anything. . . . It has made me stronger to speak out and question—I am more self-assured. And, I realize that a lot of people that I am talking to who I thought were bright, really are not—and that I am actually very bright. You know, it makes you feel differently about the way you see yourself and see others."

Davis might argue that Brenda and Tracy's comments support the idea that women who have chosen to undergo plastic surgery do not perceive themselves as passive victims or the "cultural dopes" of an oppressive, patriarchal society. Rather, they are active agents capable of negotiating their lives even under the worst of circumstances. Even though receiving breast implants caused Brenda, Tracy, and others tremendous suffering, these women were able to transform their struggles into enlightening and "empowering" experiences. I agree with this interpretation of these experiences. The women I spoke with who became educated about the risks associated with implants, and about the health problems they experienced after receiving these devices, in a sense, had become empowered, viewing themselves as active agents who had the capacity to transform a terrible ordeal into a positive experience.

However, as I have demonstrated throughout this book, the extent to which agency plays a role in women's experiences with implants is not always constant. For instance, women's descriptions of their relationships with husbands, lovers, and family members suggest that, in hindsight, women perceived their decision to seek implants not as a liberating choice, but as an action taken under specific interpersonal pressure. The feelings of regret and mixed emotions some women reported experiencing immediately following their plastic surgeries further illustrates the ambiguous nature of agency. Even though these women initially believed they were taking the right course of action to alleviate their personal suffering by undergoing plastic surgery, they explained that this suffering intensified after their surgeries. As they attempted to renegotiate their identities with a new outward physical appearance, they began to feel more like sex objects and more self-conscious about their bodies than they did before receiving their implants. Finally, women's accounts of their experiences with breast implants have shown that while some women may eventually find a positive dimension to receiving breast implants, others continue to feel powerless. In the previous chapter, for instance, I demonstrated how a woman's perception of her capacity to take charge of her life can be constrained by economic and cultural factors.[10] The women in my sample who had become angry and had taken a political stance about their implant-related troubles had, at one point in time, also felt helpless and hopeless. These women became "empowered" only after they began to educate themselves about the long-term health effects of silicone and were able to find validation for their implant-related troubles and concerns.

Thus, the degree to which "agency" accounts for women's involvement with surgery to enhance the size or shape of their breasts may vary among women, and can change over the course of one woman's experiences with breast implants. Although Davis does not explicitly make this point, her account of Irene's case implies it. Before Irene took hold of her life and became politicized, she had "closeted herself in her home," and seemed to center her life "around interaction with various doctors and unsuccessful attempts with new implants." She just "let it all happen."[11] Irene saw herself as a helpless victim of circumstance until she became fed up with her doctors and decided to educate herself about her own health problems and the potential side effects of silicone.

The women Davis interviewed were fully aware of cultural norms that shaped ideas about femininity. However, they decided to reshape their bodies anyway. They took their lives into their own hands, believing that cosmetic surgery would improve their life circumstances—and, indeed, it did. Most of Davis's respondents felt "empowered" not only because they had overcome resistance from family and friends who urged them not to undergo surgery, but also because, with their new bodies, they were able to renegotiate their identities with a new outward bodily appearance. Even those women who experienced many implant-related complications felt "empowered" because they had educated themselves about the risks associated with the devices and took pride in this accomplishment.

In the remainder of this chapter, I argue that just as perceptions of one's capacity to "take action" can vary among women and change over time so, too, can the meaning they attribute to empowerment. Davis argues that agency is "central to both why women decide to have cosmetic surgery, and how they experience its outcome." [12] Yet, in her analysis, she conflates the way a woman feels about her "choice" to undergo cosmetic surgery with the way she feels about her "choice" to take a political stance when her surgery has failed, calling each decision an "empowering" experience. In so doing, she obscures the idea that choices are made under different conditions of freedom and constraint, and that a woman's awareness of these conditions can drastically change over the course of her experiences with breast implants. "Agency," thus, is more complex than in Davis's account, since it may refer not only to a woman's self-conscious capacity to take actions to improve her life circumstances, but also to her ability to reflect back on these actions and, in the process, redefine why she had chosen to follow through with them in the first place. My respondents' implant-related experiences illustrate how agency becomes more self-conscious as women begin to develop a deeper understanding of the political, social, and cultural contexts that shape their life experiences.

In Bookman and Morgen's anthology about women activists, they argue that empowerment "begins when [women] change their ideas about the causes of their powerlessness, when they recognize the systemic forces that oppress them, and when they act to change the conditions of their lives." [13] Similarly, the women I spoke with who had decided to take their lives into their own hands and learn more about implant-related risk, did so only after beginning to link their lack of knowledge to the oppressive structure of the society in which they lived. "Empowerment" was experienced differently by these women, yet almost always involved their recognition of the larger cultural and systemic forces that influenced their decision to seek breast implants. At the time women opted to receive implants, many had believed that they were taking the best course of action to relieve their personal suffering. In hindsight, however, they came to the realization that they had been passive victims who had fallen prey to a society that places more value on a woman's outward appearance than her health. For many of them, empowerment involved reconceptualizing their sense of self as "feminine" as they began to confront the possibility of implant removal.

Opting for Removal: Becoming "More than Just Breasts"

Like the women Davis interviewed, many of my respondents were initially delighted with the results of their plastic surgeries and were glad they had made the decision to undergo surgery to enhance the size and shape of their breasts.[14] Their new breasts gave them an entirely new outlook on life, enabling them to feel more confident and self-assured about who they were in relation to how their bodies appeared.[15] However, many of these women eventually developed implant-related complications and symptoms and began to regret the decision they had made to undergo plastic surgery. They had educated themselves about the possible long-term health effects associated with breast implants and were convinced that the only option they had to alleviate their anxieties about their future health was to have their implants removed. Consequently, twenty out of the forty women in my sample chose to have this surgery to avoid developing new health problems or worsening conditions. Even though several of these women had learned that implant removal might leave them scarred and disfigured,[16] they were willing to take this chance, rather than put their health at greater risk. Mona, for instance, commented, "It is funny how much it used to mean for me to have big breasts. And, now, it means more to have my health." Similarly, Sophie explained, "Although I was having pain, I was still contemplating on keeping my implants in and putting up with them. . . . But, I got to the point where I just felt that it was useless to have beautiful breasts when you are sick. I want my health back."

In the process of deciding whether or not to have their implants removed, women had to come to terms with developing a new sense of self—but, this time, in relation to a body image they knew would be less than ideal. Just as the decision to receive breast implants involved the renegotiation of identity with a change in bodily appearance, so, too, did the decision for implant removal. In this way, both decisions can be perceived as "empowering" experiences since, in both cases, women took action to alleviate their personal suffering—women chose to have implants to feel better about their appearances, and they chose to have their implants removed to set themselves at ease about their future health.

However, a woman's decision for removal also involves her ability and willingness to recognize the larger cultural context that shaped her reasons for choosing to have breast implants in the first place. Indeed, many of the women I interviewed explained that facing the prospect of returning to a flat-chested body gave them the opportunity to reflect back on their experiences before and after receiving implants and to realize that, in fact, they had been taken in by cultural standards of femininity and female bodily appearance. Only with these insights could they redefine their own self-concept as feminine and move forward in their lives. Thus, "empowerment" is not simply about women's capacity to make choices, but also involves their ability and willingness to recognize, in hindsight, the contexts that shape these choices. For example, as Alice deliberated about her decision to have her implants removed, she began to question cultural ideals of femininity and change her own conception of self as "feminine." Only after having gone through this process did she truly feel "empowered."

Alice is a married, middle-class woman in her early forties who has lived in southern California most of her life. She is about five feet, four inches tall, slender, and has short, straight black hair, and dark-brown eyes. In hindsight, Alice realized that her reason for having breast implants was related to her unconscious desire to "relive her miserable adolescence." Growing up in a place where fair skin and blue eyes was the norm, she constantly felt insecure about her dark, Italian features: "I didn't like being so Italian-looking because I was in a high school full of these tall blondes in the late sixties, early seventies." Receiving breast implants, a face lift, and cheek implants by the time she was thirty-four, Alice believed that "this time [she would] be attractive to the guys." Although Alice initially felt "ecstatic" about her new body and felt "finally pretty enough to be out there," when she began developing implant-related health problems, "it all came crashing down." After months of joint pain, sleeplessness, hair loss, headaches, chronic fatigue, and other side effects, Alice decided to have her implants removed in 1993. She explained to me the range of emotions she experienced after making this decision:

> I cried buckets before I had the implants removed because my breasts were really beautiful. They were really, really beautiful and I did look good. It was that typical—you know, petite-little-voluptuous-playboy type of look that I had. I was just afraid of what I would look like afterwards—not knowing, be-

cause, I had remembered what I had looked like before the implants which
was flat and droopy. It was the grief and sadness of changing again—changing to possibly something that was negative and for losing what I had—what
I had gained—that little I had gained, in spite of all the illness.

Nevertheless, as Alice worked through her grief, she began to accept
the anticipated outcome of her surgery. In the process, she developed a
different understanding of "femininity" and female bodily appearances:

> I think I am looking at [femininity] now more toward a European model
> rather than an American model. The American model is perhaps more su-
> perficial, more artificial and the European model is more—I think it is more
> like being comfortable in your own skin, being happy with who you are. . . .
> There is a sense of comfort with one's own sexuality and sensuality. I think
> that is what it is—the comfort with being female which I don't think Ameri-
> can women have. . . . There is more of a softness and the ability to say, "I
> am woman and I am soft and there is no need for me to prove myself differ-
> ent by being hard and having you try to accept me because I have to put on
> a hard edge."

Through her experience of loss, grief, and body acceptance, Alice's
sense of herself as "feminine" shifted from an "American" ideal, which
she saw as artificial, superficial, and external, toward a more "Euro-
pean" ideal, which, in her mind, is characterized by more inward qualities (i.e., feeling "comfortable in your own skin"). By defining femininity in terms of these two separate and distinct models, Alice was able
to make sense of the context that shaped both her reasons for wanting
to have larger breasts, as well as her reasons for deciding to have her
breast implants removed. Having reconceptualized "femininity," she
was ready to accept her dark, Italian features and her post-implant, flat-
chested body, and she began incorporating these characteristics into a
new sense of self. Not only did Alice think differently about herself
in relation to her outward appearance, but she also felt empowered to
change her views about her life in general: "My experiences with breast
implants have changed my whole view of what I want out of life. I don't
want to have to be success-oriented or think that what I do for a living
is what is going to define me as a person, as a human being. I want to
have a lot of friends and family around me. I want to live in a society
that is not so stressed out about going to work and working, working,
working all the time without making time for pleasure, fun, people and
enjoying life."

Gayle similarly found that her decision to have her implants removed made her think about the meaning she attributed to "femininity": "I have to assume that part of what I used to consider feminine was tied up into how my body looked. Otherwise, I wouldn't have had the implants. Today, that is not where my femininity is. It is inside now. It is in my heart, in my spirituality. And, my body is just a housing for that." Just as Alice's perception of "femininity" as an inward quality, rather than an outward characteristic, led to changes in her life goals, Gayle, too, began to incorporate her new understanding of this concept into her daily life experiences: "It no longer matters what I am wearing and I find that I wear less makeup now than I ever did."

Alice, Gayle, and other women I interviewed found that their decision to have their breast implants removed enabled them to develop a deeper understanding of who they were in relation to how their bodies appeared. Knowing that this surgery might leave them permanently disfigured, they no longer chose to rely on cultural ideals of female attractiveness as a standard for measuring their own sense of self as "feminine." Instead, they began to renegotiate their identities and, in the process, were able to find richer and more fulfilling ways of thinking about their lives. Nina's perception of femininity was also transformed after she decided to have her implants removed at the age of thirty-eight: "Previously, femininity to me was more of an essence. I wasn't a living, true being, but this essence of a—I would say of a maternal, caretaker to men. I fit right into that role of being, you know, dangled on their arm, being objectified. Now, I want to own my femininity differently. . . . I just want to take more charge with who I am, which way I am going to go, what direction I am going to allow my life to flow and not be so passively led through this process." In hindsight, Nina believed that, in a sense, she had been taken in by cultural images of femininity and female bodily perfection—she had undergone surgery to have her breasts enlarged during a time in her life when she allowed herself to be "objectified" and "dangled on" the arms of men. However, after she had her implants removed, she no longer wanted to be this passive victim of oppressive stereotypes but hoped that her experiences with breast implants would enable her to "own [her] femininity differently" and "take charge" of her life. Even when her plastic surgeon suggested she undergo additional surgery to reconstruct her breasts once her implants were removed, Nina did not acquiesce to his wishes, but adamantly refused his offer: "There is part of me that gets so angry.

It's like, don't they [plastic surgeons] get this? I have had enough of being molded like this piece of putty into any shape that you want me to be or what you think looks right."

Other women I spoke with explained that they, too, refused their plastic surgeons' offers to "improve" their appearances after implant removal. For example, Sheila's surgeon wanted to replace her silicone implants with "safer" saline ones. However, she refused, exclaiming, "If I can't deal with my body for who I am at this point in my life, then I better forget about the boobs and go into deep therapy!" Similarly, Abby, who received just one implant following a mastectomy, went to her plastic surgeon to have the device removed. The surgeon agreed to perform the surgery but suggested that she undergo an additional operation so that he could transfer fatty tissue from her remaining, healthy breast to the other side of her chest. Even though Abby realized that this surgery would leave her more "symmetrical," she rejected the offer.

While these women had reached a point in their lives where they could define themselves apart from their outward appearances, they realized that their plastic surgeons remained caught up in their role as "artists," perpetuating ideals of female bodily perfection. In fact, some women said that some plastic surgeons had refused to remove their implants because they were concerned about the "cosmetic result" of this surgery.[17] Gwen, for example, was very clear that she wanted to have her implants removed, even though she knew that, in her case, a mastectomy would be necessary since her implants had ruptured and silicone had migrated into her surrounding breast tissue. Although she was no longer concerned about how her body appeared, her plastic surgeon was reluctant to perform this surgery because he was, "worried about what [Gwen] would look like." Rather than give up, Gwen took charge of this situation. She called her plastic surgeon, exclaiming: "Look, I came to see you because I was in pain and because something was wrong. . . . And you are trying to tell me that I am not going to get a perfect result—you are missing the point. The point is, something is medically wrong with me and I want it fixed and I really don't care about what I am going to look like."

Deciding whether or not to remove a woman's implants is a dilemma for plastic surgeons because it completely contradicts the goals of their practice—rather than make a woman more "beautiful," the surgery inevitably leaves women looking worse than before. Given this explanation, it makes sense that plastic surgeons refuse to perform this surgery on women because it will leave them with "undesirable" results. Yet, the way that plastic surgeons define "undesirable" is intrinsically related to their own preconception of what a woman should look like—well-proportioned or large-breasted. Many of the women I interviewed, on the other hand, had broken away from this cultural ideal of female attractiveness. After realizing that their method of achieving ideal femininity had failed, they started to question the meaning they were attributing to "beautiful breasts" and, in the process, began to develop a different self-concept as "feminine."

Confronting the possibility of returning to a flat-chested body enabled many of the women I interviewed to reflect upon the reasons why they had decided to receive breast implants and to acknowledge the possibility that they had fallen prey to cultural ideals of female beauty and femininity. These ideals were conveyed to women in different ways. For instance, while Alice gradually realized that her understanding of femininity stemmed from the blond-haired, blue-eyed environment in which she was raised, Nina felt that her conception of femininity was rooted in her relationships with men. Nevertheless, in each case, Alice, Nina, and other women I spoke with had, over time, come to believe that they had defined their sense of self as "feminine" in terms of their bodily appearances—more specifically, their breast size.

Even though women knew that implant removal would leave them scarred and possibly disfigured, they viewed their decision to do away with their breasts as empowering. They were glad that they had taken what they perceived as a necessary step toward improving their health. Moreover, they were proud that they no longer experienced the shame and embarrassment they had felt about their bodies before they had received breast implants. Frances, who had received two implants after a bilateral mastectomy, commented, "Having my implants removed didn't make me feel different—I am happy to say that I have come to a point in my life where I am more than just breasts." Sheila also explained, "I am very happy to say that I have somehow resolved my not feeling good about myself by not having bigger breasts. I am really happy with the results of my surgery. [My breast size] is back to where it was. You know, it is okay that I am not big." Sophie, too, felt empowered by her decision to have her implants removed. Prior to making this decision, she had joined a support group for women with breast implants. Not until attending her first meeting did she become aware of the possibility that "without larger breasts, you are still a woman": "I realized at the meeting, as I was looking around at all of the women who had already gone through this [ex-plantation]—who were all flat-chested—when I saw them, I said to myself, 'These are the most beautiful women I have ever seen—as well as the strongest and bravest.'" After Sophie had her implants removed, she became even more involved in the group, hoping to educate and "save innocent women who could become victims in the future."

Redefining Relationships

Sophie explained that she, too, felt as though she had been fooled by the image of "the beautiful breast," mistakenly thinking that receiving implants would save her marriage to a man who constantly ridiculed her about her "flat chest." Other women I interviewed similarly believed that their decision to have breast implants was made under specific interpersonal pressure; they had been convinced by their spouses, boyfriends, parents, or peers that they would receive more love and attention only if they changed their outward appearances.[18] However, after their surgeries, many of these respondents were dismayed to find that having larger breasts did not improve their relationships with these significant others. Moreover, when they discovered that they had agreed to a surgery that not only failed to improve their sexual and social lives, but could leave them permanently disabled and disfigured, they became terribly frightened and angry. Several of these women joined support groups where they found validation for their fears and concerns. They began to educate themselves about implant-related risk as well as their worsening health conditions and were empowered with the knowledge they had gained.

However, "empowerment" for these women was linked not only to their realization that they could be knowledgeable about health, illness, and disease causation; but also to their ability to make sense of the social contexts that shaped their decision to undergo plastic surgery in the first place. After women's surgeries had failed, many of them began to question their own sense of self in relation to their bodily attributes. In the process, those women I interviewed who felt that their decision to have their breasts enlarged had been made under specific interpersonal pressure began to question the meaning of their relationships. In effect, many decided to relinquish their ties with individuals in their lives who judged them by their appearances, and began to form new relationships with people who were less concerned about conforming to cultural standards of bodily perfection. For instance, Sophie was upset and depressed after her husband had left her for another woman. However, her feelings for him lessened after she met a man who cared for her even after she had developed debilitating symptoms and had undergone surgery to have her implants removed:

> I now have a boyfriend who loves me in spite of the fact that I am flat-chested. And, he is the best man I have met in my life. He took care of me after my operation [to have her implants removed]. He took me into his home when I had no place to go and was too ill to look for a place to live. Very few men would have done that for me. They would expect something in return right away. And, he can't even touch me after the surgery. You know, before, I thought that femininity had a lot to do with looks—big breasts, shapely. Now I realize that a man can still love me and still see me as a woman without these characteristics.

For Sophie, finding a more meaningful intimate relationship coincided with developing a different sense of herself as "feminine." Once, she defined femininity in terms of outward appearances; however, her new relationship enabled her to realize that "it is the person inside that counts."

Similarly, after Gayle finally decided to have her implants removed after experiencing months of constant fatigue and aching joints, she realized that she had "come to a place in [her] life where [she was] not her body." She further stated, "If someone doesn't want to be with me—an intimate, sexual companion doesn't want to be with me because I have small breasts and scars—if they don't want to be with me because of that, then I don't want to be with that person."

Other women explained that their experiences with breast implants enabled them not only to become more accepting of their own bodies, but also more accepting of, and willing to relate to, men whose outward appearances did not reflect cultural ideals of male attractiveness. Rose, for instance, felt that her ex-husband had pressured her into having breast implants. When she began to experience autoimmune-related symptoms, she became angry that he had been so concerned about the way she looked but, at the same time, admitted, "I, too, used to be guilty of judging people based on their appearance." Reflecting on her life without larger breasts, she commented, "Maybe through all these experiences [with implants], people will learn a little compassion and maybe take the time to find out what a person is really like. I mean, I used to see a man and think, 'He's not really good-looking.' And, now I would talk to him and he might be the nicest man in the world. And, boy, you ought to see some of the men I talk to today—they're fat, they're bald—but, you know, I am developing a lot of new friends out of all of this. I think it is a humbling experience."

While many women found that their experiences with breast implants enabled them to transform the meaning of their relationships with men, other women discovered that these experiences empowered them to redefine their friendships with women. For instance, when I met Patty, she still had her implants but had made an appointment with a plastic surgeon to have them removed after learning that the symptoms she was experiencing—aching joints, stomach irritability, and chronic fatigue—could be related to these devices. She explained that making this decision was difficult, but at the same time, it gave her a new perspective on life. Part of her new outlook involved making new friends: "Well, the friends I have now are no longer the catty ones. The kind of friends I used to have—they wanted to make sure they looked better than you and dressed better than you and drive a better car than you. I learned that that doesn't give you a very good rapport for a friendship. Now, I have picked friends who I feel comfortable with— who I feel I don't have to be better than." Patty's old friendships perpetuated her belief that the only way to improve life circumstances is to change outward appearances: "I thought that if I got implants, my life would be better, if I grew my hair long, my life would be better." Only after confronting the possibility that her implants were making her sick and facing the fact that she might need to have them removed, did she begin to understand that she had "never looked inside to see who [she] really was." Despite all of the problems she had experienced with her implants, she nevertheless believed, "From what I have gone through, I think I can help people a lot more. And, I have a lot more fulfillment and substance in my life than I would have had if I kept on being 'Mrs. Fufu' with implants and going to New York City to get my hair done. I have a bit more balance."

Tracy also said that after she had her implants removed, she relinquished her friendships with certain women. She told me about one "ex-friend" who, after noticing the reduction in Tracy's chest size, seemed more interested "in the size of [her] breast cup" than how Tracy was feeling about her surgery. Rather than comfort and console Tracy, she gossiped about Tracy's experiences with implants to other women in her community. After this incident, Tracy began to think about the nature of her friendships with women, and she has come to perceive her experiences with implants as "symbolic" for how she has redefined these relationships: "*These* [my implants] are poison—*she* [her old friend] was poison. I don't want to be surrounded by, and will not let myself be surrounded by, people who are negative, vicious types of people. These people are not allowed to be in my life. If I find them, I get rid of them very quickly. To think that she should be more concerned with the size of my breasts than she was about how I felt. . . . I don't want to be with people like that, I just don't. Now I pick and choose." Even though Patty and Tracy did not explicitly link their decision to undergo surgery to enhance the size of their breasts with their relationships with female peers, their comments, nevertheless, indicate that their friendships had perpetuated ideals of female bodily appearance, possibly leading them to plastic surgeons' offices. Only after they experienced troubles with their implants did they begin to question the influence these relationships had over their lives and reach the decision that they no longer wanted to maintain friendships with women who paid more attention to outward appearances than personal attributes.

Many of the women I interviewed explained that their interpersonal relationships had no influence over their decision to have breast implants. For instance, most of the women I interviewed who had undergone reconstructive surgery following mastectomies explained that their reasons for having their breast(s) reconstructed had more to do with their desire to appear more "normal," than a need to feel more "feminine." These women did not elect to have surgery to satisfy their husbands, boyfriends, or peers; rather, they wanted to eliminate the anticipated stigma of a "diseased-looking," breastless body.[19] Nevertheless, even some of these women described how their experiences with breast implants compelled them to examine their interpersonal relationships and, in effect, question the meaning of their own sense womanhood. Brenda, for instance, at the age of fifty, decided to end her thirty-year marriage to "a man who could not psychologically take much in life," because he was unable to cope with her implant-related complications and symptoms. As Brenda's health deteriorated after receiving implants, she not only became acutely aware of her husband's inability to respond to her problems but also began to question her own role in their relationship:

> It is odd to say that you can lose yourself in a long-term marriage, and rearing your children. . . . A woman who is in the age bracket that I fall in, and is from the lifestyle that I came from, who has not had the experiences that

young people have who are going into higher education and having life experiences and several relationships—women like myself are conditioned to be a
support system and not to expect from life what younger people would. I was
brought up a certain way—to marry and stay married—and that was that.
So, consequently, I expected this spouse to support me. And, when that didn't
happen, that was just one more thing to deal with.

Brenda did not choose simply to "deal with" her husband's behavior.
Rather, she began to think about the larger social context shaping her
relationship with her husband and, in the process, began to question
cultural expectations of womanhood.

When Brenda married in the early 1960s, the ideology of separate
gender spheres was still in full force. In this era, men were assumed to
be the primary financial providers for their families, while their wives
were perceived as passive, docile homemakers who took care of the children and provided emotional support for their husbands.[20] After Brenda
took notice of her husband's reluctance to cross over these gendered
boundaries to take care of and comfort her when she became ill, Brenda
began to question her own expected role as dutiful wife. In the process, she decided to develop new strategies for coping with her implant-
related troubles. Rather than passively continue in a relationship that
made her feel trapped and isolated, Brenda took charge of her life—she
asked her husband for a divorce and found a psychologist to provide her
with the emotional support that her husband never offered.

Even though Brenda believed that her experiences with breast implants instigated problems in her marriage, she perceived these experiences as the catalyst enabling her to transform her identity: "An experience such as the one I have been through can make you a stronger
person. It can make you watch out for and question other aspects of
your life that you ordinarily had great respect for and would not question—such as my marriage. I am now actively involved with the divorce—actively participating in it. I am questioning what these lawyers are doing, why they are doing it. Because, this type of experience
[with breast implants] makes you this type of person. It makes you more
responsible."

Transformations in Health Care Decision Making

The women I interviewed had turned to plastic surgery to provide them
with a quick, simple, and safe solution for improving their bodily appearances. Women like Brenda, who had breast implants following a

mastectomy, explained that they were basically in a "state of shock" after discovering they had breast cancer, and were willing to accept any solution their doctors had to offer to alleviate their fears and anxieties associated with losing their breast(s). When Brenda's surgeon recommended reconstructive surgery with implants, without hesitation, she "went along with it, trusting the medical community." The women I spoke with who decided to have their breasts enlarged with implants also trusted their doctors. They never doubted their plastic surgeons' ability to reshape their bodies and never considered the possibility that these doctors might provide them with misleading and inaccurate information. All of my respondents reasonably assumed that physicians are knowledgeable about the risks involved with the devices they use and the procedures they perform. Moreover, they presumed that medicine itself is a certain and precise science capable of curing—not compounding—people's health-related troubles.

However, women's assumptions about physicians and their expectations of medicine changed throughout the course of their experiences with breast implants. Most of my respondents reported experiencing numerous health problems and complications that they attributed to their implants. As their health worsened, they visited many different doctors, hoping to find assurance and validation for their troubles. Instead, they found resistance and avoidance—most of their physicians were unwilling to acknowledge a possible relationship between silicone and disease and continually minimized and dismissed women's health problems and concerns. In effect, most of the women I spoke with increasingly became disillusioned with medicine and began to doubt the abilities of medical "experts": How could their plastic surgeons have assumed that inserting a plastic bag full of silicone inside a woman's body would not lead to any damaging side effects? And, if their poor health was not related to their implants, why were other physicians unable to come up with alternative explanations for the strange symptoms they were experiencing?

In the process of asking these and similar types of questions, the meaning of expertise for these women gradually changed as their perception of authority shifted from those who were supposed to be knowledgeable based on their professional status, to themselves.[21] Rather than continue to place their faith in medicine, many of my respondents decided to educate themselves about implant-related risk and join support groups and information networks to better understand how their breast implants were affecting their lives. In the process, they gained more confidence in themselves, realizing their own capacity to understand complicated medical explanations and evaluate scientific reports, which either supported or denied a relationship between implants and disease. These women discovered that their experiences with implants enabled them to transform their identities, from passive patients who had assumed that medicine was capable of providing complete and accurate information about disease causation, to health care activists who acknowledged the possibility that medical knowledge is fallible. Empowerment, for these women, occurred as they began to accept responsibility for their own health care decisions and help other women become better-informed consumers of medical care.

Eve explained that she "used to depend on the medical profession to make [her] diagnosis and [to] treat." This line of reasoning had guided all of her health care decisions, including her decision to have breast implants: After giving birth to her son, she felt miserable about the appearance of her breasts and turned to a plastic surgeon to "fix" her problems. However, shortly after her surgery, she began to experience debilitating rheumatic symptoms and a number of other health problems. After listening to news reports detailing the possible long-term health effects of silicone breast implants, she was certain that her implants were causing her troubles. Yet, when she visited her physicians and articulated these concerns, they dismissed her concerns, telling her that the scientific studies about implant-related risk are inconclusive. Realizing that she could no longer rely on these doctors for assurance, Eve joined a national support and information network for women with implants and started to conduct her own research on the health effects of breast implants. She went to the library and photocopied newspaper clippings and medical and scientific journal articles, and wrote to various health care organizations asking for information. Eve took pride in her ability to educate herself, boasting about her basement full of boxes packed with implant-related literature. In short, her experiences with implants enabled her to develop an entirely new way of thinking about her health care: "Now, I depend on myself to make my diagnosis. I do my research to find out how I should be treated and then I find a physician who will do that. I kind of manage my own care now."

Rose, who became an active member of a support group for implant recipients, described a similar course of action as she became increasingly convinced that her implants were connected to her worsening health. She explained that prior to her troubles with implants, "I always had been one who, in no way, would hurt my doctor's feelings by going to another doctor for a second opinion. I just was not brought up to do that kind of thing." But, during the course of her experiences with breast implants, she started to realize that doctors do not always possess complete and accurate knowledge about health and illness: "I really think that everybody needs to know that doctors are not God and that it is okay that you ask questions and that you insist on second opinions. . . . I wouldn't hesitate to ask for a second, or even a third opinion now. People also need to know that they can go to a library and do their own research. There is a wealth of information that people have access to." Sheila also felt that women should take a more activist stance toward managing their health care. She was angry and upset with the FDA and the medical community for turning their backs on women's implant-related troubles. But, she also believed that women could learn from the implant disaster and accept more of the responsibility for what they decide to do to their bodies: "The implant disaster was all about money—that is never going to change. But, I think we need to get the message across that women know what [the medical community, implant manufacturers, and the government] are doing. We also have to stop letting them do it to us. When you go to the doctor's office—they can put whatever they want on the market, and we take it. We have to learn to say 'No!'"

Rose, Sheila, and other women I spoke with came to the realization that medical knowledge is frequently uncertain and that physicians are capable of making mistakes. Their experiences with implants enabled them to question their own expectations of medicine and medical expertise and, in the process, learn that they were capable of developing their own theories about disease causation and educating themselves about their own health conditions. Although they continued to rely on their doctors for diagnosis and treatment of their implant-related symptoms, they had developed a more holistic approach toward managing their care, which balanced their own ideas about health and illness with their physicians' biomedical reasoning. Many women also incorporated alternative or self-help treatments into their health care regimens. For instance, Alice began to visit a massage therapist and practice reflexology to alleviate the pain in her joints, and Gloria began taking various vitamins to "repair [her] damaged tissues and cells" caused by her Sjögren's syndrome. These women discovered that the more they learned about their own health conditions and the side effects associated with breast implants, the more they could educate other implant recipients. Gloria, for instance, started her own support group in which she and other women with implants discussed various therapies and remedies for treating their implant-related symptoms. Rose explained that even her plastic surgeon now turns to her for information about breast implants: "We did not like each other at first. But, I do give him a lot of credit. He took it upon himself to read the literature I gave him, and he went to some of the lectures on implants I told him about. Finally, he said to me, 'You know, I think you have a point here.' Basically, he was man enough to say that he was wrong. And, from that point on, he made a point to become more informed. In fact, a few months back, he asked my personal opinion about saline implants, and so I gave him some documentation on the harmful effects of these implants. He read it and now he no longer implants women with saline or silicone."

However, Rose reported that other doctors she visited were not as receptive to listening to her own perspectives on health, illness, and disease causation. Instead, these physicians "get angry, thinking you are trying to self-diagnose." In fact, many of the women I interviewed explained that while they viewed their new activist stance toward managing their health care as "empowering," their physicians perceived the change in their behavior as confrontational and defiant.[22] For example, even though Alice had taken charge of her health care decisions, her doctors did not seem to appreciate her new approach: "Doctors don't like me because I bring in a list of questions, and I ask them questions that sort of pin them against the wall sometimes and it makes them feel uneasy. . . . They feel like, 'Oh here is this woman, she is threatening my ego, and who does she think she is . . . she is going to be one of those difficult or noncompliant patients.'" Implicit in Alice's remark is the idea that "noncompliance" is subjectively defined and interpreted in accordance with physicians' expectations of appropriate patient behavior.[23] In this way, noncompliance can be viewed as "an ideology that assumes and justifies medical authority."[24] Alice realized that physicians were presumed to possess more knowledge about health and illness than their patients, and she understood that the difficult questions she posed to her own doctors about her implant-related health conditions were viewed as a threat to their medical expertise. Thus, in her mind, the more involved she became in her health care decisions, the more she was perceived as a "difficult" patient. Nevertheless, she felt empowered as she developed a new sense of confidence in her capacity to take charge of her health care decisions: "In this two-and-a-half-year process of being sick and seeing so many doctors, and being betrayed by them—coming up against situations with these doctors where I know more than they do in some respects, and having them telling me that they know more about my body—when they are not living in it. . . . In this process, I have learned that I have to be responsible for my own body."

Before receiving implants, many women assumed that plastic surgeons and other medical experts could provide them with simple and safe solutions to all of their health-related problems. However, as they came to the realization that their implants could be related to their debilitating health conditions, they began to acknowledge the possibility that medical knowledge is incomplete and, sometimes, inaccurate. In a sense, these women felt as though they had been duped by cultural myths about medicine as a "true" and "accurate" discipline, and fooled by the image they had of their physicians as "Gods." But, at the same time, their recognition of these false ideals empowered them to challenge the unbalanced relationship between their physicians and themselves.

According to the women in this study, empowerment does not simply involve a feeling of personal growth, but, even more so, it entails a recognition of the larger structural, cultural, and systemic forces that shape their life experiences. The power of hindsight allowed the women I spoke with to question the system of beliefs that shaped their understandings of femininity, as well as their expectations of medicine and science. As women became more conscious of the cultural conditions that constrained and limited the ways in which they thought about health, illness, and the female body, they gradually came to the realization that their decision to receive breast implants had less to do with agency, or their ability to take charge of their lives, than with their own subordinate role in society. These women believed that, in a sense, they had been the passive victims of ideological manipulation—they falsely assumed that their sexual and social lives would improve if they adhered to a cultural standard of femininity, that medical experts could provide them with a safe and simple solution for improving their poor self-images, and that medical and scientific knowledge is accurate, complete, and certain. Once these women recognized the fallibility of these assumptions, they could rethink the logic that guided their life decisions and develop richer, more fulfilling ways of thinking about their lives. Patty explained:

I have begun to realize that there has to be something better than this little glass bubble of a world. And, the way I describe it—it is like, if you go searching for these material things all your life (and, I think my implants were a part of this), these things to make you look better—you are never going to find what you are truly searching for. And, you can have as much money in the world and you could still have that void in your soul. Someone described this feeling once as standing against a telephone pole and the wind whipping and going right through you. That was the best description that I had ever heard. It was. You could be in a room with a million people and feel so alone. I used to look at other people and wonder what it would be like to be just like them, to be everybody else but me. . . . That is so sad—to want to be anybody else but yourself. That is exactly how I used to go through life. . . . But, after what I have been through, I don't think I would ever feel like that today.

Perhaps the greatest lesson to be learned by the women who participated in this study is that without an awareness of the prevailing system of beliefs that shape individual behaviors and actions, we can not begin to understand and ameliorate the problems embedded within the structure of modern medicine.

Notes

Chapter One

1. For purposes of confidentiality, I have changed the names of all the women who participated in this study, as well as the names of their family members, physicians, attorneys, and friends.

2. I discuss how these symptoms prevented Jenna from carrying on with her daily activities in Chapter 4.

3. Susan Brownmiller, *Femininity* (New York: Linden Press/Simon and Schuster, 1984), 40.

4. Iris Young, *Throwing Like a Girl and Other Essays in Feminist Philosophy and Social Theory* (Bloomington: Indiana University Press, 1990), 189.

5. American Society of Plastic and Reconstructive Surgeons, Position Statement, 1982.

6. The details of this settlement are discussed in Chapter 2.

7. Eugene Kaw, "Medicalization of Racial Features: Asian American Women and Cosmetic Surgery," *Medical Anthropology Quarterly* 7 (1993): 74–89.

8. Ralph Cook, Robert Delongchamp, Maryann Woodbury, Laura Perkins, and Myron Harrison, "The Prevalence of Women with Breast Implants in the United States—1989," *Journal of Clinical Epidemiology* 48 (1995): 519–25.

9. Sherine Gabriel, Michael O'Fallon, C. Mary Beard, Leonard Kurland, John Woods, and L. Joseph Melton III, "Trends in the Utilization of Silicone Breast Implants, 1964–1991, and Methodology for a Population-Based Study of Outcomes," *Journal of Clinical Epidemiology* 48 (1995): 527–37.

10. Cook et al., "The Prevalence of Women with Breast Implants," 519–25; Marcia Angell, "Breast Implants—Protection or Paternalism?" editorial, *New England Journal of Medicine* 326 (1992): 1695–98.

11. Gabriel et al., "Trends in the Utilization of Silicone Breast Implants," 527–37.

12. In fact, one support group leader edited my announcement before placing it in her group's newsletter. She changed the wording so that it read: "Doctoral student . . . wishes to interview women who experience *problems* with breast implants." I did not interview women who responded to this announcement. Never-

theless, I am not certain how other support group leaders presented my research to members of their groups. Even though my announcement addressed all women with breast implants, leaders who viewed my research as a vehicle for politicization may have intentionally tried to recruit women who experienced problems with these devices.

13. Marcia Angell, *Science on Trial: The Clash of Medical Evidence and the Law in the Breast Implant Case* (New York: W. W. Norton, 1996).

14. For instance, see Charles Rosenberg, "The Silicone Papers," review of *Science on Trial: The Clash of Medical Evidence and the Law in the Breast Implant Case*, by Marcia Angell. *New York Times* (book review section), July 14, 1996; and Annetine C. Gelijns and Alan Moskowitz, "Derelictions," *Science* 273 (1996): 917.

15. The most comprehensive of these sites is "United Silicone Survivors of the World" at *ussw.trimaris.com*. For an ongoing discussion of women's responses to the latest information regarding breast implants see "Breast Implants: Reader Feedback" at *www.everywoman.com/now/implant.htm*; "Breast Implants" at *www.compuvar.com/internet/implants.html*; and the breast implant message board available through the Better Health and Medical Network at *www.betterhealth.com*.

16. I conducted most of my interviews in the privacy of women's own homes. However, when the respondent's home was not a convenient or private place to talk, we would meet in a quiet coffee shop or nearby park.

17. Ann Oakley, "Interviewing Women: A Contradiction in Terms," in *Doing Feminist Research*, edited by Helen Roberts (Boston: Routledge and Kegan Paul, 1981), 30–60.

18. Ibid., 49.

19. The average length of the interviews was about two hours, although one interview was less than an hour long and a few were close to four hours long. Although I had a prepared interview schedule, I made an effort to ask women open-ended questions so that they could talk about their implant-related experiences with minimal interruption. This narrative approach is a common method used in qualitative sociology. See, for example, Catherine Kohler Riessman, *Narrative Analysis* (Newbury Park: Sage Publications, 1993). Medical sociologists and anthropologists particularly have found the approach useful for understanding how patients make sense of their illnesses in relation to larger social and cultural contexts, in addition to how they interpret their experiences with health care providers. For instance, see Arthur Kleinman, *The Illness Narratives* (New York: Basic Books, Inc., 1988); Garreth Williams, "The Genesis of Chronic Illness: Narrative Reconstruction," *Sociology of Health and Illness* 6 (1984): 176–200; and Susan Bell, "Becoming a Political Woman: The Reconstruction and Interpretation of Experience through Stories," in *Gender and Discourse: The Power of Talk*, edited by Alexandra Dundas Todd and Sue Fisher (Norwood: Ablex Publishing Corp., 1988), 97–123.

Chapter Two

1. The number of women who have received implants is difficult to determine since surgeons have tended to base their estimates on the frequency of surgical procedures, and implant manufacturers' estimates are based on the number of devices,

which often include inventories and presurgical breakage. In either case, implant replacements, ruptures, and removals are not taken into account. Despite these discrepancies, most recent estimates suggest that the number is closer to one million than two million. For instance, see Ralph Cook, Robert Delongchamp, Maryann Woodbury, Laura Perkins, and Myron Harrison, "The Prevalence of Women with Breast Implants in the United States—1989," *Journal of Clinical Epidemiology* 48 (1995): 519–25; and Mary Beth Terry, Mary Louise Skovron, Samantha Garbers, Elizabeth Sonnenschein, and Paolo Toniolo, "The Estimated Frequency of Cosmetic Breast Augmentation among US Women, 1963 through 1988," *American Journal of Public Health* 85 (1995): 1122–24.

2. Marcia Angell, "Breast Implants—Protection or Paternalism?" editorial, *New England Journal of Medicine* 326 (1992): 1695–98.

3. Angela Bonavoglia, "Alternatives: Know the Risks," *Ms.* 6 (1996): 58.

4. With this method, doctors insert a steel tube into the navel, channel it underneath the skin of the rib cage until it reaches the breast region. An empty silicone sac is pushed through the tube then filled with salt water. The tube is then removed from the body. The procedure leaves only a faint scar at the site of the navel incision.

5. John Byrne, *Informed Consent: A Story of Personal Tragedy and Corporate Betrayal* (New York: McGraw-Hill, 1996), 178.

6. Marc Lappé, *Chemical Deception: The Toxic Threat to Health and the Environment* (San Francisco: Sierra Club Books, 1991).

7. Ibid., 156.

8. Herbert Conway and Dicran Goulian, "Experience with an Injectable Silastic RTV as a Subcutaneous Prosthetic Material," *Plastic and Reconstructive Surgery* 32 (1963): 294–302.

9. Philip Hilts, "Silicone: Friend or Foe? Strange History of Silicone Held Many Warning Signs," *New York Times*, Jan. 18, 1992.

10. Byrne, *Informed Consent*, 41.

11. Ibid., 42.

12. Ibid., 41.

13. Human Resources and Intergovernmental Relations Subcommittee of the Committee on Governmental Operations, *The FDA's Regulation of Silicone Breast Implants* (Washington, D.C.: Government Printing Office, 1993).

14. Byrne, *Informed Consent*, 42–43.

15. Walter Peters and Dennis Smith, "Ivalon Sponge Prostheses: Evaluation of 19 Years after Implantation," *Plastic and Reconstructive Surgery* 67 (1981): 514–18.

16. M. T. Edgerton and A. R. McClary, "Augmentation Mammaplasty: Psychiatric Implications and Surgical Indications," *Plastic and Reconstructive Surgery* 21 (1958): 279–305.

17. A. W. Schwartz and J. B. Erich, "Experimental Study of Polyvinyl-formula (Ivalon) Sponge as a Substitute for Tissue," *Plastic and Reconstructive Surgery* 25 (1960): 1.

18. B. S. Oppenheimer, E. T. Oppenheimer, and A. P. Stout, "Sarcomas Induced in Rodents by Embedding Various Plastic Films," *Proceedings of the Society for Experimental Biology and Medicine* 79 (1952): 366.

19. Conway and Goulian, "Experience with an Injectable Silastic RTV as a Subcutaneous Prosthetic Material," 294.

20. Ibid.

21. Ibid., 301.

22. Edgerton and McClary, "Augmentation Mammaplasty."

23. Ibid., 301.

24. Ibid., 297.

25. Ibid., 298.

26. Howard Updegraff and Karl Menninger, "Some Psychoanalytic Aspects of Plastic Surgery," *American Journal of Surgery* 25 (1934): 554–58.

27. Ibid., 557.

28. G. G. Hay, "Psychiatric Aspects of Cosmetic Nasal Operations," *British Journal of Psychiatry* 116 (1970): 85–97.

29. G. Hill and G. Silver, "Psychodynamic and Aesthetic Modifications for Plastic Surgery," *Psychosomatic Medicine* 12 (1950): 345.

30. W. E. Jacobson, M. T. Edgerton, E. Meyer, A. Canter, and R. Slaughter, "Psychiatric Evaluation of Male Patients Seeking Cosmetic Surgery," *Plastic and Reconstructive Surgery* 26 (1960): 356.

31. M. T. Edgerton, E. Meyer, and W. E. Jacobson, "Augmentation Mammaplasty: Further Surgical and Psychiatric Evaluation," *Plastic and Reconstructive Surgery* 27 (1961): 279–302.

32. Ibid., 301.

33. I discuss the definition of a "good candidate" in further detail in Chapter 3.

34. Byrne, *Informed Consent*, 41.

35. Ibid., 41–42.

36. Even though Dow Corning Corporation applied for a Notice of Claimed Investigational Exemption for a New Drug (IND) for facial injections in 1965, breast augmentation with injections was not even permitted in the study because of the known medical complications and risks (Human Resources and Intergovernmental Relations Subcommittee of the Committee on Governmental Operations, *The FDA's Regulation of Silicone Breast Implants*).

37. Byrne, *Informed Consent*, 44.

38. Ibid., 46.

39. Ibid.

40. Lappé, *Chemical Deception*, 158.

41. Ibid., 158.

42. Ibid., 159.

43. For a more detailed description of different types of breast implants, see Nancy Bruning, *Breast Implants: Everything You Need to Know*, 2d ed. (Alameda, Calif.: Hunter House, 1995).

44. Joan E. Rigdon, "Saline Implants Now Seem to Carry Health Hazards as Well," *Wall Street Journal*, Feb. 4, 1993.

45. U.S. Dept. of Health and Human Services, *HHS News*, Jan. 5, 1993.

46. Women who had their breasts enhanced with the sponge in the 1950s experienced the same problem. Although many physicians discontinued using the im-

plantable sponge because women's breasts became so hard, they did not follow the same course of action with the breast implant.

47. Human Resources and Intergovernmental Relations Subcommittee of the Committee on Governmental Operations, *The FDA's Regulation of Silicone Breast Implants.*

48. Frank Vasey and Josh Feldstein, *The Silicone Breast Implant Controversy: What Women Need to Know* (Freedom, Calif.: The Crossing Press, 1993).

49. Thomas Burton, "How Industrial Foam Came to Be Employed in Breast Implants," *Wall Street Journal,* Mar. 25, 1992.

50. R. Guidon, M. Therrien, C. Rolland, M. King, J. L. Grandmaison, S. Kaliaguine, P. Blais, H. Pakdel, and C. Roy, "The Polyurethane Foam Covering the Meme Breast Prosthesis: A Biomedical Breakthrough or a Biomaterial Tar Baby?" *Annals of Plastic Surgery* 28 (1992): 342–353.

51. Burton, "How Industrial Foam Came to Be Employed in Breast Implants."

52. Vasey and Feldstein, *The Silicone Breast Implant Controversy.*

53. Lappé, *Chemical Deception.*

54. Prior to this case, most of the suits against implant manufacturers had been strictly product liability cases and were quietly settled out of court for relatively small sums of money (between $30,000 and $75,000); see Byrne, *Informed Consent.*

55. Health Facts, "Silicone Breast Implants: Serious Problems are Virtually Guaranteed" (New York: Center for Medical Consumers Inc., Dec. 1989), 4–6.

56. Philip Hilts, "Company to Release Data Questioning Implant Safety," *New York Times,* Jan. 23, 1992.

57. Human Resources and Intergovernmental Relations Subcommittee of the Committee on Governmental Operations, *The FDA's Regulation of Silicone Breast Implants.*

58. Dow Document, May 16, 1975.

59. Dow Document, Jan. 15, 1976.

60. Human Resources and Intergovernmental Relations Subcommittee of the Committee on Governmental Operations, *The FDA's Regulation of Silicone Breast Implants.*

61. B. F. Uretsky, J. J. O'Brien, E. H. Courtiss, et al., "Augmentation Mammaplasty Associated with a Severe Systemic Illness," *Annals of Plastic Surgery* 3 (1979): 445–49.

62. Dow Document, Jan. 15, 1976.

63. Human Resources and Intergovernmental Relations Subcommittee of the Committee on Governmental Operations, *The FDA's Regulation of Silicone Breast Implants.*

64. Ibid.

65. Ibid., 17–21.

66. *Federal Register,* 53 (Jun. 24, 1988): 23,856–77.

67. Human Resources and Intergovernmental Relations Subcommittee of the Committee on Governmental Operations, *The FDA's Regulation of Silicone Breast Implants,* 5.

68. Personal correspondence with a friend of Hopkins, 1993.

69. David Kessler, "The Basis of the FDA's Decision on Breast Implants," *New England Journal of Medicine* 326 (1992): 1713–15.

70. See, for example, Burton, "How Industrial Foam Came to Be Employed in Breast Implants"; Burton, "Breast Implants Raise More Safety Issues," *Wall Street Journal*, Feb. 4, 1993; Reuters, "Dow Corning Cites Subpoena for Falsified Implant Data," *Boston Globe*, Feb. 18, 1993; Hilts, "Company to Release Data Questioning Implant Safety"; and Hilts, "Silicone: Friend or Foe?"

71. Human Resources and Intergovernmental Relations Subcommittee of the Committee on Governmental Operations, *The FDA's Regulation of Silicone Breast Implants*.

72. Before Mariann Hopkins was awarded over $7 million, fewer than two hundred cases were pending against this manufacturer for health care claims.

73. Gina Kolata, "3 Breast Implant Makers Agree to Pay $3.7 Billion," *New York Times*, Feb. 20, 1994.

74. Byrne, *Informed Consent*, 234.

75. In some cases, women were able to sue Dow Chemical, which had participated with Dow Corning in conducting early safety studies of silicone; see Byrne, *Informed Consent*, 235–36.

76. See Judith Graham, "Increased Offer on Implants Assailed: Dow Corning Would Pay Out $2.4 Billion in Settlement," *Chicago Tribune*, Aug. 26, 1997. For further details of this new proposal, see Gina Kolata, "Dow Corning Seeks to Settle Implant Case," *New York Times*, Aug. 26, 1997.

77. The epidemiological literature on implant-related risk is covered in Chapter 6.

78. The literature on implant-related risk is reviewed in the *Federal Register*, Jan. 8, 1993, 58: 3438–39.

79. *Federal Register*, Jan. 8, 1993, 58: 3438.

80. Ibid.

81. See Vasey and Feldstein, *The Silicone Breast Implant Controversy*.

82. Sherine Gabriel, John Woods, Michael O'Fallon, Mary Beard, Leonard Kurland, and Joseph Melton III, "Complications Leading to Surgery after Breast Implantation," *New England Journal of Medicine* 336 (1997): 677–82.

83. H. Hayes, M. S. Vandergrift, and W. C. Diner, "Mammography and Breast Implants," *Plastic and Reconstructive Surgery* 82 (1988): 1–6.

84. *The Federal Register*, Jan. 8, 1993, 58: 3438–39.

85. Human Resources and Intergovernmental Relations Subcommittee of the Committee on Governmental Operations, *The FDA's Regulation of Silicone Breast Implants*.

86. Jack Fisher, "The Silicone Controversy—When Will Science Prevail?" *New England Journal of Medicine* 326 (1992): 196–98.

87. Marcia Angell, "Breast Implants—Protection or Paternalism?"

88. Yauo Kumagai, Yuichi Shiokawa, Thomas Medsger Jr., and Gerald Rodnan, "Clinical Spectrum of Connective Tissue Disease after Cosmetic Surgery," *Arthritis and Rheumatism* 27 (1984): 1–12.

89. Ibid., 1.

90. Vasey and Feldstein, *The Silicone Breast Implant Controversy*.

91. See, for example, Y. Okano, M. Nishikai, and A. Sato, "Scleroderma, Primary Biliary Cirrhosis, and Sjögren's Syndrome after Breast Augmentation with Silicone Injection: A Case Report of Possible Adjuvant Disease," *Annals of Rheumatic Disorders* 43 (1984): 520–22; W. Kaiser, G. Biesenbach, U. Stuby, P. Grafinger, and J. Zazgornik, "Human Adjuvant Disease: Remission of Silicone Induces Autoimmune Disease after Explantation of Breast Augmentation," *Annals of Rheumatic Disorders* 49 (1990): 937–38; J. O. Naim, R. J. Lanzafame, J. C. Van Oss, "The Adjuvant Effect of Silicone-Gel on Antibody Formation in Rats," *Immunological Investigations* 22 (1993): 151–61; and R. M. Silver, E. E. Sahn, A. J. Allen, S. Sahn, W. Greene, J. C. Maize, and P. D. Garen, "Demonstration of Silicon in Sites of Connective-Tissue Disease in Patients with Silicone Gel Breast Implants," *Archives of Dermatology* 129 (1993): 63–68.

92. See H. Spiera, "Scleroderma after Silicone Augmentation Mammoplasty," *Journal of the American Medical Association* 260 (1988): 236–38; Alan Bridges, Carol Conley, Grace Wang, David Burns, and Frank Vasey, "A Clinical Immunological Evaluation of Women with Silicone Breast Implants and Symptoms of Rheumatic Disease," *Annals of Internal Medicine* 118 (1993): 929–36.

93. See B. O. Shoaib, B. M. Patten, and D. S. Caulkin, "Adjuvant Breast Disease: An Evaluation of 100 Symptomatic Women with Breast Implants or Silicone Fluid Injections," *Keio Journal of Medicine* 43 (1992): 79–87; R. F. Spierra, A. Gibofsky, and H. Spiera, "Silicone Gel-Filled Breast Implants and Connective Tissue Disease: An Overview," *Journal of Rheumatology* 21 (1994): 239–45; E. Giltay, H. Moens, A. Riley, and R. Tan, "Silicone Breast Prostheses and Rheumatic Symptoms: A Retrospective Follow-up Study," *Annals of Rheumatic Disorders* 53 (1994): 194–96; and Charles Hennekens, I-Min Lee, Nancy Cook, Patricia Herbert, Elizabeth Karlson, Fran LaMotte, JoAnn Manson, and Julie Buring, "Self-Reported Breast Implants and Connective Tissue Diseases in Female Health Professionals: A Retrospective Cohort Study," *Journal of the American Medical Association* 275 (1996): 616–21.

94. M. J. Duffy and J. E. Woods, "Health Risks of Failed Silicone Gel Breast Implants," *Plastic and Reconstructive Surgery* 94 (1994): 295–99; Sherine Gabriel, Michael O'Fallon, C. Mary Beard, Leonard Kurland, John Woods, and L. Joseph Melton III, "Trends in the Utilization of Silicone Breast Implants, 1964–1991, and Methodology for a Population-Based Study of Outcomes," *Journal of Clinical Epidemiology* 48 (1994): 527–37; W. Peters, E. Keystone, K. Snow, L. Rubin, and D. Smith, "Is There a Relationship between Autoantibodies and Silicone-gel Implants?" *Annals of Plastic Surgery* 21 (1994): 5–7; and K. E. Wells, C. W. Cruse, J. L. Baker, S. M. Daniel, R. A. Stern, C. Newman, M. J. Seleznick, F. B. Vasey, S. Brozana, and S. E. Albers., "The Health Status of Women Following Cosmetic Surgery," *Plastic and Reconstructive Surgery* 93 (1994): 907–12; and C. Dugowson, J. Daling, T. Koepsell, L. Voight, and J. Nelson, "Silicone Breast Implants and Risk for Rheumatoid Arthritis," *Arthritis and Rheumatism* 35 (1992): 66. The study conducted by Gabriel et al. did find a significant relationship between breast implants and reports of morning stiffness.

95. S. B. Cohen and R. J. Rohrich, "Evaluation of the Patient with Silicone Gel Breast Implants and Rheumatic Complaints," *Plastic and Reconstructive Surgery*

94 (1994): 120–25. It is interesting that the authors of this study see bias as affecting only their patients' point of view and not the viewpoints of physicians or researchers.

96. See, for example, M. Potter, S. Morrison, F. Wiener, K. X. Zhang, and F. Miller, "Induction of Plasmacytomas with Silicone Gel in Genetically Susceptible Strains of Mice," *Journal of the National Cancer Institute* 86 (1994): 1058–65; and Sydney Salmon and Robert Kyle, "Silicone Gels, Induction of Plasma Cell Tumors, and Genetic Susceptibility in Mice: a Call for Epidemiological Investigation of Women with Silicone Breast Implants," *Journal of the National Cancer Institute* 86 (1994): 1040–41.

97. C. Paletta, F. X. Paletta Jr., and F. X. Paletta Sr., "Squamous Cell Carcinoma Following Breast Augmentation," *Annals of Plastic Surgery* 29 (1992): 425–29.

98. D. M. Deapen, M. C. Pike, J. T. Casagrande, and G. S. Brody, "The Relationship between Breast Cancer and Augmentation Mammaplasty: An Epidemiological Study," *Plastic and Reconstructive Surgery* 77 (1986): 361–67; J. Y. Petit, M. G. Lee, H. Mouriesse, M. Rietjens, P. Gill, G. Contesso, and A. Lehmann, "Can Reconstruction with Gel-Filled Silicone Implants Increase the Risk of Death and Second Primary Cancer in Patients Treated by Mastectomy for Breast Cancer?" *Plastic and Reconstructive Surgery* 94 (1994): 115–19; Hans Berkel, Dale Birdsell, and Heather Jenkins, "Breast Augmentation: A Risk Factor for Breast Cancer?" *New England Journal of Medicine* 326 (1992): 1649–53; Arnold Engel, Steven Lamm, and Sheghan Lai, "Human Breast Sarcoma and Human Breast Implantation," *Journal of Clinical Epidemiology* 48 (1995): 539–44; Robert Morgan and Maryellen Elcock, "Artificial Implants and Soft Tissue Sarcomas," *Journal of Clinical Epidemiology* 48 (1995): 545–49; Dennis Deapen and Garry Brody, "Augmentation Mammaplasty and Breast Cancer: A Five Year Update of the Los Angeles Study," *Journal of Clinical Epidemiology* 48 (1995): 551–56.

99. Berkel et al., "Breast Augmentation."

100. J. J. Levine and N. T. Ilowite, "Scleroderma-like Esophageal Disease in Children Breast-fed by Mothers with Silicone Breast Implants," *Journal of the American Medical Association* 271 (1994): 213–16.

101. S. S. Teuber and M. E. Gershwin, "Autoantibodies and Clinical Rheumatic Complaints in Two Children of Women with Silicone Gel Breast Implants," *International Archives of Allergy and Immunology* 103 (1994): 105–8.

102. American Society of Plastic and Reconstructive Surgeons, Position Statement, 1992.

103. La Leche League International, *Nursing with Breast Implants*, 1992.

Chapter Three

1. Peter Conrad, "Medicalization and Social Control," *Annual Review of Sociology* 18 (1991): 211.

2. Ibid., 211.

3. Catherine Kohler Riessman, "Women and Medicalization: A New Perspective," *Social Policy* 14 (1983): 3–18.

4. For further analysis of women's involvement with plastic surgery, see Diana

Dull and Candace West, "Accounting for Cosmetic Surgery: The Accomplishment of Gender," *Social Problems* 38: 54–95.

5. Kathy Davis, "Remaking the She-Devil: A Critical Look at Feminist Approaches to Beauty," *Hypatia* 6 (1991): 21–43; Kathy Davis, "Cultural Dopes and She-Devils: Cosmetic Surgery as Ideological Dilemma," in *Negotiating at the Margins: The Gendered Discourses of Power and Resistance*, edited by Kathy Davis and Sue Fisher (New Brunswick, N.J.: Rutgers University Press, 1993), 23–47; and Kathy Davis, *Reshaping the Female Body: The Dilemma of Cosmetic Surgery* (New York: Routledge, 1995).

6. Davis, "Cultural Dopes and She-Devils," 30.

7. Davis, *Reshaping the Female Body*, 157.

8. See, for example, Marcia Millman, *Such a Pretty Face: Being Fat in America* (New York: Norton, 1980); Nancy Baker, *The Beauty Trap: Exploring Woman's Greatest Obsession* (New York: Franklin Watts, 1984); Susan Brownmiller, *Femininity* (New York: Linden Press/Simon and Schuster, 1984); and Wendy Chapkis, *Beauty Secrets: Women and the Politics of Appearance* (Boston: South End Press, 1986).

9. See, for example, Alison Jaggar and Susan Bordo, eds., *Gender/Body/Knowledge* (New Brunswick, N.J.: Rutgers University Press, 1989); and Mary Jacobus, Evelyn Fox Keller, and Sally Shuttleworth, *Body/Politics: Women and the Discourses of Science* (New York: Routledge, 1990).

10. Davis, "Cultural Dopes and She-Devils," 24.

11. Susan Bordo, *Unbearable Weight: Feminism, Western Culture, and the Body* (Berkeley and Los Angeles: University of California Press, 1993).

12. Michel Foucault, *Discipline and Punish* (New York: Vintage Books, 1979).

13. Bordo, *Unbearable Weight*, 31.

14. Ibid., 31–32.

15. Ibid., 32.

16. Ibid., 31.

17. Ibid., 31.

18. Ibid., 20.

19. Dull and West, "Accounting for Cosmetic Surgery," 54–95.

20. Davis, "Remaking the She-Devil."

21. Brownmiller, *Femininity*, 16.

22. Rita Freedman, *Beauty Bound* (Lexington, Mass.: Lexington Books, 1986), 67.

23. Dull and West, "Accounting for Cosmetic Surgery," 62.

24. Dull and West offer this same line of thought.

25. Dull and West, "Accounting for Cosmetic Surgery."

26. Ibid., 63.

27. Irving Zola, "Bringing Our Bodies and Ourselves Back In: Reflections on a Past, Present, and Future Medical Sociology," *Journal of Health and Social Behavior* 32 (1991): 1–16.

28. Miriam Schwartz, "A Sociological Reinterpretation of the Controversy over 'Unnecessary Surgery,'" *Research in the Sociology of Health Care* 3 (1984): 194.

29. American Society of Plastic and Reconstructive Surgeons, Position Statement, 1992.

30. In fact, two of the women in the sample of forty (Sarah and Gloria) did not

even know whether their surgery was considered "reconstructive" or "cosmetic." These cases are described in the Introduction under the heading "Experiences and Methodology."

31. See Schwartz, "A Sociological Reinterpretation of the Controversy over 'Unnecessary Surgery.'"

32. The majority of women I interviewed who had breast cancer were diagnosed with this illness more than ten years ago (see Table 1.2 in Introduction). In effect, women's concerns about breast implants took precedence over their concerns about the recurrence of cancer during the course of the interviews.

33. Audre Lorde, *The Cancer Journals* (San Francisco: Spinsters Ink, 1980).

34. Iris Young, *Throwing Like a Girl and Other Essays in Feminist Philosophy and Social Theory* (Bloomington: Indiana University Press, 1990), 204.

35. Delese Wear, "'Your Breasts/Sliced Off': Literary Images of Breast Cancer," *Women and Health* 20 (1993): 81–100.

36. Beth Meyerowitz, Shelly Chaiken, and Laura Clark, "Sexual Roles and Culture: Social and Personal Reactions to Breast Cancer," in *Women with Disabilities: Essays in Psychology, Culture and Politics*, edited by Michelle Fine and Adrienne Asch (Philadelphia: Temple University Press, 1988), 80.

37. Lorde, *The Cancer Journals*, 42.

38. Meyerowitz et al., "Sexual Roles and Culture," 80.

39. Young, *Throwing Like a Girl*, 204.

40. Ibid.

41. Lorde, *The Cancer Journals*, 64.

42. Ibid., 61.

43. Ruth Merkatz, Grant Bagley, and Jane McCarthy, "A Qualitative Analysis of Self-Reported Experiences among Women Encountering Difficulties with Silicone Breast Implants," *Journal of Women's Health* 2 (1993): 106.

44. David Hidalgo, "Breast Reconstruction," in *Women Talk about Breast Surgery: From Diagnosis to Recovery*, edited by Amy Gross and Dee Ito (New York: Harper Perennial, 1990), 251.

45. Young, *Throwing Like a Girl*, 204.

46. This is a major difference between the women who had breast implants for cosmetic reasons and those who had implants for reconstructive purposes.

Chapter Four

1. Kathy Davis, *Reshaping the Female Body: The Dilemma of Cosmetic Surgery* (New York: Routledge, 1995).

2. I address how women responded to learning about the risks associated with their implants in Chapter 5.

3. Davis, *Reshaping the Female Body*, 157.

4. Ibid., 138.

5. Ibid., 156.

6. Ibid., 139.

7. See Introduction for discussion of my recruitment strategy and the representativeness of my sample. The women Davis interviewed for her follow-up study were all white and most came from working-class to middle-class backgrounds.

The women ranged in age from seventeen to forty-three years old. Some of these women were employed outside the home, while others were full-time housewives. Davis conducted her study in the Netherlands, where cosmetic surgeries are covered by national health insurance. This may account for the class difference between our two samples. Since health insurance in the United States does not cover cosmetic surgery, only those who can afford to undergo it do so.

8. Davis, *Reshaping the Female Body*, 104–14.

9. This was particularly the case for women who received breast implants for perceived "cosmetic" reasons. Women who chose to have implants after a mastectomy or to correct for some other type of "disfigurement" are apt to perceive their reconstructive surgery as a means of restoring their identity. For instance, women who have had mastectomies are replacing a part of their body that was surgically removed and want to appear "like themselves" again. On the other hand, women who have breast implants to enlarge their breasts are, in essence, creating new identities. (All of the women in Kathy Davis's study had implants for cosmetic reasons.)

10. Wendy Chapkis, *Beauty Secrets: Women and the Politics of Appearance* (Boston: South End Press, 1986), 3.

11. Davis, *Reshaping the Female Body*.

12. Ibid., 163.

13. Some women's symptoms were less evident than others. For instance, some women had rashes across their faces (indicating signs of lupus), or looked flushed and worn out. However, other women appeared quite healthy despite their reports of debilitating fatigue and aching joints. (For example, see Jenna's story in the Introduction.)

14. Christine now suspects that all of these symptoms are a result of an autoimmune response to her implants. Other women have mentioned allergic-type reactions to alcohol and various types of food, as well as memory loss. Christine suspects that the spot on her labia is the result of lymphocytes having migrated to this area.

15. All three of the women I interviewed who had implants after the age of fifty attributed their arthritis, aching joints, and other symptoms to "growing old." In fact, Maureen and Kate continue to adhere to the medical profession's opinion that breast implants are "perfectly safe." Brenda, is the only one of these three women who has come to the understanding that her symptoms are more implant-related than age-specific.

16. I provide a more detailed analysis of physicians' tendency to "psychologize" women's implant-related troubles in Chapter 6.

17. Joseph Schneider and Peter Conrad discuss the disclosure or concealment of illness (specifically, epilepsy) in terms of being "in the closet" or "out of the closet." Individuals use the strategy of being "in the closet" with their illness (if it can be hidden) to prevent "others from applying limiting and restrictive rules that disqualify one from normal social roles." Employment, therefore, tends to be an area where being "in the closet" has its advantages. Schneider and Conrad argue that the door to the closet is revolving, allowing individuals to negotiate when and where to disclose or conceal their illness; see Joseph Schneider and Peter Conrad, "In the Closet with Illness: Epilepsy, Stigma Potential and Information Control," *Social Problems* 28 (1980): 32–44.

18. Symptoms associated with Sjögren's syndrome include dry eyes, burning, decreased tearing, redness, itching, eye fatigue, increased sensitivity to light, and low-grade fevers. Symptoms associated with scleroderma include swelling and puffiness of the fingers or hands, arthritis involving small joints of the hands, skin thickening, and bowel problems; see Robert Shmerling and Matthew Liang, "Laboratory Evaluation of Rheumatic Diseases," *Primer on the Rheumatic Diseases* (Atlanta: The Arthritis Foundation, 1993).

19. Davis, *Reshaping the Female Body*.

20. Ibid., 156.

21. Ibid., 157.

22. Ibid., 151.

Chapter Five

1. Letters from patients to the FDA also support this claim; see Human Resources and Intergovernmental Relations Subcommittee of the Committee on Governmental Operations, *The FDA's Regulation of Silicone Breast Implants* (Washington, D.C.: Government Printing Office, 1993).

2. Implant mammaplasty is indeed a big business, one of the most frequently performed plastic surgeries in the United States, costing women and insurance companies between $1,000 to $3,000 per procedure.

3. Roberta Apfel and Susan Fisher conducted a study on women's responses to the health effects of DES and similarly found that women exposed to the drug wanted to know who the "villains" were behind the story. Many blamed their physicians, the pharmaceutical industry, and the FDA for prescribing, producing, and permitting the marketing of a drug that was harmful to exposed women and children. The authors argue against the label "villains," as well as a conspiracy theory, suggesting that greed and profits tell only a small part of the story; see Roberta Apfel and Susan Fisher, *To Do No Harm: DES and the Dilemmas of Modern Medicine* (New Haven: Yale University Press, 1984).

4. See, for example, Howard Waitzkin, *The Second Sickness: Contradictions of Capitalist Health Care* (New York: Free Press, 1983); Howard Waitzkin, "A Critical Theory of Medical Discourse: Ideology, Social Control, and the Processing of Social Context in Medical Encounters," *Journal of Health and Social Behavior* 30 (1990): 220–39; and Paul Starr, *The Social Transformation of American Medicine* (New York: Basic Books, 1982).

5. Alexandra Dundas Todd, *Double Vision: An East-West Collaboration for Coping with Cancer* (Hanover, N.H.: University Press of New England, 1994), 119.

6. For examples, see Todd, *Double Vision*, 119.

7. Ibid., 120.

8. Ibid., 121.

9. For example, see Alexandra Dundas Todd, *Intimate Adversaries: Cultural Conflict Between Doctors and Women Patients* (Philadelphia: University of Pennsylvania Press, 1989); and Sue Fisher, *In the Patient's Best Interest: Women and the Politics of Medical Decisions* (New Brunswick, N.J.: Rutgers University Press, 1986).

10. Using DES and hormonal replacement therapy, Susan Bell has written extensively on this issue; see Susan Bell, "A New Model of Medical Technology De-

velopment: A Case Study of DES," *Research in the Sociology of Health Care* 4 (1986): 1–32; Susan Bell, "Technology in Medicine: Development, Diffusion, and Health Policy," in *Handbook of Medical Sociology*, edited by Howard Freeman and Sol Levine (Englewood Cliffs, N.J.: Prentice Hall. 1989), 185–204; Susan Bell, "Gendered Medical Science: Producing a Drug for Women," *Feminist Studies* 21 (1995): 469–500; and Susan Bell, "Technology Assessment, Outcome Data and Social Context: The Case of Hormone Therapy," in *Getting Doctors to Listen: Ethics and Outcomes Data in Context*, edited by P. Boyle (Washington, D.C.: Georgetown University Press, 1997).

11. Emily Martin, *Flexible Bodies: Tracking Immunity in American Culture—From the Days of Polio to the Age of AIDS* (Boston: Beacon Press, 1994).

12. Ibid., 245.

13. Ibid., 245.

14. Bell, "Gendered Medical Science," 471.

15. Rita agreed to let me take the brochure, make a copy, then return it to her.

16. Dow Brochure, "Facts You Should Know About Your New Look," 1976.

17. Susan Bordo, *Unbearable Weight: Feminism, Western Culture and the Body* (Berkeley and Los Angeles: University of California Press, 1993), 250–51.

18. See Chapter 2.

19. Dow Brochure, 1.

20. Ibid., 1.

21. Ibid., 2.

22. Ten of the forty women I interviewed had received one or two implants following mastectomies. Out of these ten women, six reported that they had never actively questioned their surgeons about implant safety. The other four women who had had mastectomies were extremely cautious about their decision to get implants and asked their surgeons numerous questions regarding the safety of the devices.

23. One woman I spoke with who had undergone the same procedure, but on both sides of her chest, had referred to herself as "Frankenstein," as two valves surrounded by scar tissue stuck out on each side of her chest. I found her description quite ironic since her implants were intended to make her "look beautiful."

24. Brenda also told me that her insurance company did not cover the reconstruction of her nipple, which to Brenda seems quite ironic since she was born with her nipple, but not the mound of fatty breast tissue she developed later in life. Her experience with her insurance company again reinforces the cultural idea that the "size" of breasts—or how they appear to onlookers—is their most important physical characteristic.

25. Also see Chapter 3.

26. Linda Cook, Janet R. Daling, Linda F. Voigt, M. Patricia DeHart, Kathleen E. Malone, Janet L. Stanford, Noel S. Weiss, Louise A. Brinton, Marilie D. Gammon, and Donna Brogan, "Characteristics of Women With and Without Breast Augmentation," *Journal of the American Medical Association* 277 (1997): 1612–17.

27. Ibid., 1616.

28. Throughout my interview with Carmen, I became increasingly uncomfortable with her lack of knowledge around implant-related risk, especially since I had already interviewed women who had saline implants who were experiencing health

problems believed to be related to the device. Since I saw my role as "researcher," and not as "informant," and since there is so much uncertainty around this issue, I chose to provide information to my respondents only when they asked. The information I gave to women was in the form of names and addresses of support groups and information networks for women with breast implants. Occasionally, if women asked about other women's experiences with implants and their health problems, I would talk to them about what I had heard, without revealing the identities of other respondents. (For details about how I addressed this dilemma of interviewing refer to the methodology section in my Introduction.)

29. Along with breast implants, there are similar cases of drugs that have not been approved by the FDA and yet are widely used. For example, the FDA has never recommended the use of progestin in hormonal replacement therapy for menopausal or postmenopausal women, nevertheless, physicians regularly prescribe it for this purpose; see Bell, "Technology Assessment, Outcome Data and Social Context: The Case of Hormone Therapy." I suspect that most women taking this drug are not aware of this fact.

30. Human Resources and Intergovernmental Relations Subcommittee of the Committee on Governmental Operations, *The FDA's Regulation of Silicone Breast Implants*, 35.

31. Ibid.

32. Ibid.

33. Ibid.

34. For a review of this literature see, for example, Bell, "Technology Assessment, Outcome Data and Social Context."

35. Bell, "Technology Assessment, Outcome Data and Social Context."

36. Human Resources and Intergovernmental Relations Subcommittee of the Committee on Governmental Operations, *The FDA's Regulation of Silicone Breast Implants*.

37. Ibid., 39.

38. Ibid., 38.

39. Ibid., 41.

40. Ibid., 40.

41. Ibid.

42. This finding completely diverges from findings presented in Kathy Davis's analysis; see Davis, *Reshaping the Female Body*.

43. Human Resources and Intergovernmental Relations Subcommittee of the Committee on Governmental Operations, *The FDA's Regulation of Silicone Breast Implants*, 40.

44. Barbara Katz Rothman, *In Labor: Women and Power in the Birthplace* (New York: W. W. Norton, 1991), 33.

45. See Chapter 4.

Chapter Six

1. This show aired on December 10, 1990.

2. In the early 1990s, scientific reports suggested that closed capsulotomies can cause implants to rupture or leak; see Jill Leibman, Marjorie Kossoff, and Beth D.

Kruse, "Intraductal Extension of Silicone from a Ruptured Breast Implant," *Plastic and Reconstructive Surgery* 89 (1992): 546–47.

3. See Chapter 2 for a review of literature on the risks associated with polyurethane-covered implants.

4. See, for example, Yauo Kumagai, Yuichi Shiokawa, Thomas Medsger Jr., and Gerald Rodnan, "Clinical Spectrum of Connective Tissue Disease after Cosmetic Surgery," *Arthritis and Rheumatism* 27 (1984): 1–12; Y. Okano, M. Nishikai, and A. Sato., "Scleroderma, Primary Biliary Cirrhosis, and Sjögren's Syndrome after Breast Augmentation with Silicone Injection: A Case Report of Possible Adjuvant Disease," *Annals of Rheumatic Disorders* 43 (1984): 520–22; and L. P. Endo, N. L. Edwards, S. Longley, L. C. Corman, R. S. Panush, "Silicone and Rheumatic Diseases," *Seminars in Arthritis and Rheumatism* 17 (1987): 112–18.

5. Frank Vasey and Josh Feldstein, *The Silicone Breast Implant Controversy: What Women Need to Know* (Freedom, Calif.: Crossing Press, 1993).

6. Deborah Gordon, "Tenacious Assumptions in Western Medicine," in *Biomedicine Examined*, edited by Margaret Lock and Deborah Gordon (Boston: Kluwer Academic Publishers, 1988), 32.

7. Elliot Mishler, "Critical Perspectives on the Biomedical Model," in *Social Contexts of Health, Illness, and Patient Care*, edited by Elliot Mishler, Lorna Amara Singham, Stuart Hauser, Ramsay Liem, Samuel Osherson, and Nancy Waxler (New York: Cambridge University Press, 1981), 1.

8. Ibid., 1. There has been resistance to this belief within certain medical settings. For example, Harvard University's Pathways Program, which began in 1984, was designed to overcome assumptions about physicians as distant and detached from their patients by encouraging medical school students to combine "the best qualities of the skillful and caring physician"; see Byron Good and Mary-Jo Delvecchio Good, "'Learning Medicine': The Construction of Knowledge at Harvard Medical School," in *Knowledge, Power and Practice*, edited by Shirley Lindenbaum and Margaret Lock (Berkeley: University of California Press, 1993), 85.

9. Emily Martin, *The Woman in the Body: A Cultural Analysis of Reproduction*, 2d ed. (Boston: Beacon Press, 1992), 20.

10. Ibid.

11. Alison Jaggar, *Feminist Politics and Human Nature* (Sussex, Eng.: Harvester Press, Ltd., 1983): 316.

12. Anne Fausto-Sterling, *Myths of Gender: Biological Theories about Women and Men* (New York: Basic Books, 1992).

13. Ibid., 121.

14. Alexandra Dundas Todd, "Women's Bodies as Diseased and Deviant," *Research in Law, Deviance, and Social Control* 5 (1983): 84.

15. Martin, *The Woman in the Body*.

16. Vander et al., quoted in Martin, *The Woman in the Body*, 45.

17. Susan Bell, "Changing Ideas: The Medicalization of Menopause," *Social Science and Medicine* 24 (1987): 535–42.

18. Susan Bell, "Becoming a Political Woman: The Reconstruction and Interpretation of Experience through Stories," in *Gender and Discourse: The Power of Talk*, edited by Alexandra Dundas Todd and Sue Fisher (Norwood: Ablex Publishing Corp, 1988), 97–123.

19. Diethylstilbestrol, or DES, is a drug that was developed in 1938 and used for over thirty years to prevent pregnancy complications in women. It was later linked to reproductive problems and a rare form of vaginal cancer in the daughters of women who took the drug.

20. Ibid., 107.

21. J. Wallen, "Physician Stereotypes about Female Health and Illness," *Women and Health* 4 (1979): 135–46; Alexandra Dundas Todd, *Intimate Adversaries: Cultural Conflict Between Doctors and Women Patients* (Philadelphia: University of Pennsylvania Press, 1989); Sue Fisher, *In the Patient's Best Interest: Women and the Politics of Medical Decisions,* (New Brunswick, N.J.: Rutgers University Press., 1986).

22. Barbara Ehrenreich and Deirdre English, *For Her Own Good: 150 Years of the Experts' Advice to Women* (New York: Doubleday, 1989).

23. Adele Clarke, "Women's Health: Life-Cycle Issues," in *Women, Health, and Medicine in America,* edited by Rima Apple (New York: Garland Publishing, Inc., 1990), 28.

24. Elaine Showalter, "Victorian Women and Insanity," in *Madhouses, Mad-Doctors, and Madmen: The Social History of Psychiatry in the Victorian Era,* edited by Andrew Scull (Philadelphia: University of Pennsylvania Press, 1981), 54.

25. Graham John Barker-Benfield, *The Horrors of the Half-Known Life: Male Attitudes toward Women and Sexuality in 19th Century America* (New York: Harper Row, 1976).

26. Sheryl Ruzek, "Feminist Visions of Health: An International Perspective," in *What Is Feminism?* edited by Ann Oakley and Juliet Mitchell (New York: Pantheon Books, 1986), 184–207.

27. For more on the medicalization of childbirth, see Barbara Katz Rothman, *In Labor: Women and Power in the Birthplace* (New York: W. W. Norton, 1991).

28. Henry Frank, "Violence Against Women: The Pharmaceutical Industry," *Free Inquiry in Creative Sociology* 15 (1987): 199–205.

29. The Dalkon Shield was implicated in numerous cases of pelvic inflammatory disease, spontaneous septic abortions and eighteen cases of death; see Morton Mintz, *At Any Cost: Corporate Greed, Women and the Dalkon Shield* (New York: Pantheon Books, 1985); the first birth control pills were associated with dangerous conditions, including blood clots, liver disease, hypertension, cancer, diabetes, and severe depression; see Barbara Seaman and Gideon Seaman, *Women and the Crisis of Sex Hormones* (New York: Rawson Associates Publishers Inc., 1977). For discussions on the complications associated with DES, see Roberta Apfel and Susan Fisher, *To Do No Harm: DES and the Dilemmas of Modern Medicine* (New Haven: Yale University Press, 1984).

30. For discussions on the social construction of premenstrual syndrome, see Amanda Rittenhouse, "The Emergence of Premenstrual Syndrome as a Social Problem," *Social Problems* 38 (1991): 412–25; and Joan Chrisler and Karen Levy, "The Media Construct of a Menstrual Monster," *Women and Health* 16 (1990): 89–104.

31. Fausto-Sterling, *Myths of Gender.*

32. For instance, Sheila's first gynecologist, who diagnosed her with "bad PMS," was a woman.

33. For a review of this literature see Candace West, "Reconceptualizing Gender in Physician-Patient Relationships," *Social Science and Medicine* 36 (1993): 57–66.

34. Sherine Gabriel, Michael O'Fallon, Leonard Kurland, Mary Beard, John Woods, and Joseph Melton, "Risk of Connective Tissue Disease and Other Disorders after Breast Implantation," *New England Journal of Medicine* 330 (1994): 1702.

35. Arnold Engel, Steven Lamm, and Sheghan Lai, "Human Breast Sarcoma and Human Breast Implantation," *Journal of Clinical Epidemiology* 48 (1995): 539–44.

36. Robert Morgan and Maryellen Elcock, "Artificial Implants and Soft Tissue Sarcomas," *Journal of Clinical Epidemiology* 48 (1995): 545–49.

37. Dennis Deapen and Garry Brody, "Augmentation Mammaplasty and Breast Cancer: A Five Year Update of the Los Angeles Study," *Journal of Clinical Epidemiology* 48 (1995): 551–56.

38. Marc Hochberg, Robyn Miller, and Fredrick Wigley, "Frequency of Augmentation Mammoplasty in Patients with Systemic Sclerosis: Data from the Johns Hopkins–University of Maryland Scleroderma Center," *Journal of Clinical Epidemiology* 48 (1995): 565–69.

39. John Goldman, Jesse Greenblatt, Ron Joines, Leslie White, Bruce Aylward, and Steven Lamm, "Breast Implants, Rheumatoid Arthritis, and Connective Tissue Disease in a Clinical Practice," *Journal of Clinical Epidemiology* 48 (1995): 571–82.

40. For instance, the Mayo Clinic study was supported by grants from the Plastic Surgery Educational Foundation (see Gabriel et al., "Risk of Connective Tissue Disease and Other Disorders after Breast Implantation"), and two other studies were partially funded by Dow Corning Corporation; see Goldman et al., "Breast Implants, Rheumatoid Arthritis, and Connective Tissue Disease in a Clinical Practice"; and Charles Hennekens, I-Min Lee, Nancy Cook, Patricia Herbert, Elizabeth Karlson, Fran LaMotte, JoAnn Manson, and Julie Buring, "Self-Reported Breast Implants and Connective Tissue Diseases in Female Health Professionals: A Retrospective Cohort Study," *Journal of the American Medical Association* 275 (1996): 616–21.

41. Two of three authors of a study that found no evidence of a relationship between silicone and rheumatic disorders were consultants to law firms (see J. Sanchez-Guerro, P. H. Schur, and M. H. Liang, "Silicone Breast Implants and Rheumatic Disease," *Arthritis and Rheumatism* 37 [1994]: 158–68). Daniel Haney discusses this possible bias; see Daniel Haney, "Medical Editor's Role as Expert Paid by Lawyers is Scrutinized," *Boston Globe*, Dec. 12, 1994.

42. See Harold Garfinkle and Egon Bittner, " 'Good' Organizational Reasons for 'Bad' Clinical Records," in *Studies in Ethnomethodology*, edited by Harold Garfinkle (Englewood Cliffs, N.J.: Prentice Hall, 1967). Moreover, Nigel Gilbert and Christian Heath assert that physicians create medical records in order to assess and manage illness. Because these documents are not intended to be used for research purposes, inevitable biases will arise when their contents are analyzed; see Nigel Gilbert and Christian Heath, "Text, Competence and Logic: An Exercise," *Qualitative Sociology* 9 (1986): 215–236.

43. Evelyn Fox Keller, *Secrets of Life and Death: Essays on Language, Gender and Science* (New York: Routledge, 1992), 5.

44. Hennekens et al., "Self-Reported Breast Implants and Connective Tissue Diseases in Female Health Professionals."

45. Ibid., 621.

46. See Delores Kong, "Breast Implant Study Finds Some Risk," *Boston Globe,* Feb. 28, 1996.

47. Gina Kolata, "Study Cites Small Risks for Women From Breast Implants," *New York Times,* Feb. 28, 1996.

48. Wolfe's criticism of these studies was reported in the *New York Times;* see Kolata, "Study Cites Small Risks for Women From Breast Implants."

49. Hennekens et al., "Self-Reported Breast Implants and Connective Tissue Diseases in Female Health Professionals."

50. The likelihood of false positive or false negative laboratory test results may compound implant recipients' troubles. For instance, estimates suggest that prevalence of false positives produced by the most frequently ordered test in the evaluation of persons with suspected rheumatic disease (rheumatoid factor), may be as high as 25 percent. Furthermore, in a sizable subset of patients with rheumatoid arthritis, the rheumatoid factor may be negative; see Robert Shmerling and Matthew Liang, "Laboratory Evaluation of Rheumatic Diseases," *Primer on the Rheumatic Diseases* (Atlanta: The Arthritis Foundation, 1993).

51. Vasey and Feldstein, *The Silicone Breast Implant Controversy.*

52. Lappé's research suggests that silicone triggers an overstimulation of the immune system that can lead to disease; see Marc Lappé, "Silicone-Reactive Disorder: A New Autoimmune Disease Caused by Immunostimulation and Superantigens," *Medical Hypothesis* 41 (1993): 348–52.

53. Marc Lappé, *Evolutionary Medicine* (San Francisco: Sierra Club Books, 1994), 9.

54. Ibid., 10.

55. See, for example, Phil Brown and Edwin Mikkelsen, *No Safe Place: Toxic Waste, Leukemia, and Community Action* (Berkeley: University of California Press, 1990). Just as the symptoms associated with breast implants are vague and difficult to place into medical categories so, too, are the symptoms associated with various forms of environmental disease.

56. Since my interviews with Sheila and Brenda, a study has been published that indicates that scientists are beginning to find a way to diagnose and potentially validate implant recipients symptoms. Using an anti-polymer antibody (APA) assay, researchers at Tulane and Louisiana State Universities found a correlation between silicone exposure and immune system disruption. The assay detected high counts of anti-polymer antibodies in implant recipients who exhibited severe systemic symptoms, but who did not necessarily meet the criteria for specific autoimmune diseases; see Scott Tenenbaum, Janet Rice, Luis Espinoza, Marta Cuéllar, Douglas Plymale, Davis Sander, Linda Williamson, Allyson Haislip, Oscar Gluck, John Tesser, Less Nogy, Kathleen Stribrny, Julie Bevan, and Robert Garry, "Use of Anti-Polymer Assay in Recipients of Silicone Breast Implants," 349 *Lancet* (1997): 449–54. The results of this study support the notion that silicone implant recipients may

be experiencing a new type of syndrome characterized by a number of debilitating symptoms. Also see B. G. Silverman, S. L. Brown, R. A. Bright, R. G. Kaczmarek, J. B. Arrowsmith-Lowe, and D. A. Kessler, "Reported Complications of Silicone Gel Breast Implants: An Epidemiological Review," *Annals of Internal Medicine* 124 (1996): 744–56.

57. Marcia Angell, *Science on Trial: The Clash of Medical Evidence and the Law in the Breast Implant Case* (New York: W. W. Norton, 1996).

58. Ibid., 110.

59. Ibid., 152.

60. Ibid., 152–53.

61. Ibid., 209.

62. Gina Kolata, "Implant Lawsuits Create a Medical Rush to Cash In," *New York Times*, Sept. 9, 1995.

63. Richard Wronski, "Rheumatologists See No Danger in Silicone Devices," *Chicago Tribune*, Oct. 26, 1995; and Gina Kolata, "Proof of Breast Implant Peril Is Lacking, Rheumatologists Say," *New York Times*, Oct. 25, 1995.

64. "Why Judges Must Fight Bad Science: Big Settlement in Silicone Implant Cases Reveals Problem," editorial, *Los Angeles Times*, June 28, 1995.

65. Gina Kolata, "Judge Rules Breast Implant Evidence Invalid," *New York Times*, Dec. 19, 1996.

66. Nearly a quarter of the 749 women studied had implant-related complications serious enough to require further surgery. The most common complication reported is capsular contracture, followed by implant rupture, hematoma, and infection; see Sherine Gabriel, John Woods, Michael O'Fallon, Mary Beard, Leonard Kurland, and Joseph Melton III, "Complications Leading to Surgery after Breast Implantation," *New England Journal of Medicine* 333 (1997): 677–82.

67. Thomas Burton, "Frequency of Reoperations for Women with Breast Implants Put at Nearly Twenty-five Percent," *Wall Street Journal*, Mar. 6, 1997.

68. This show aired on May 14, 1997.

69. Refer to my Introduction under the heading "Experiences and Methodology" for a description of how I went about collecting data for this follow-up study.

70. See, for instance, "Breast Implants: Reader Feedback," at *www.every woman.com/how/implant2.htm*; "Breast Implants," at *www.compuvar.com/internet/implants.html*; and the breast implant message board available through the Better Health and Medical Network at *www.betterhealth.com*.

71. See "Comments from Our Guests," at *www.compuvar.com/internet/com ments.html*.

72. Kathy Keithley-Johnson, "Victims of Faulty Breast Implants Fight Enemies Within, Without," *Columbia Daily Tribune*, Mar. 11, 1997.

73. Marilyn Lloyd, "The Real Tragedy Behind Silicone Breast Implants," *Chicago Tribune*, Nov. 9, 1995.

74. Mary Vaughan, "A Head-on Collision with 'Junk Science,'" *Chicago Tribune*, Apr. 3, 1997.

75. This message was posted on April 10, 1997, on a message board accessible through the Better Health and Medical Network at *www.betterhealth.com*.

Chapter Seven

1. See Chapters 5 and 6.

2. Also see C. Wright Mills, *The Sociological Imagination* (New York: Oxford University Press, 1959).

3. In Anne Witte Garland's collection of stories about women activists, she similarly states: "Women activists point to anger as a principal motivation underlying their thinking and their behavior. Anger is often at the center of their transformations from private actors in restricted universes to public leaders in universes encompassing all the important issues of the day"; see Anne Witte Garland, *Women Activists: Challenging the Abuse of Power* (New York: Feminist Press at the City University of New York, 1988), xvii.

4. Project Impact, *Impact!* (newsletter), Apr. 1995. For a detailed criticism of this legislation see Lucinda Finley, Statement presented before the Subcommittee on Courts and Administrative Practice of the Committee on the Judiciary of the United States Senate on S.687—The Product Liability Fairness Act, 103d Congress, 2nd Sess., 1994.

5. Elliot Mishler, *The Discourse of Medicine: Dialectics of Medical Interviews* (Norwood: Ablex Publishing. Corp., 1984).

6. Phil Brown, "Popular Epidemiology and Toxic Waste Contamination: Lay and Professional Ways of Knowing," *Journal of Health and Social Behavior* 33 (1992): 267–81.

7. Phil Brown and Edwin Mikkelsen, however, suggest that within the voice of medical science, epidemiologists and clinical researchers may interpret evidence differently. For instance, some researchers choose to rely on type II errors (false negatives), rather than type I errors (false positives); "that is, they would prefer falsely to deny an association between variables when there is one than to claim an association when there is none." Other researchers tend to err on the safe side of false positives (they would prefer to assume that disease causation exists, even if it does not); see Brown and Mikkelsen, *No Safe Place: Toxic Waste, Leukemia, and Community Action* (Berkeley: University of California Press, 1990), 134. Thus, there is even more complexity involved than a straightforward dichotomy between two "voices" or "ways of knowing" suggests.

8. Although the cancer was found in Rebecca's right breast, she decided to have both breasts removed.

9. Also see Chapter 6.

10. For a compelling analysis of the expansion of scientific rationality into medical practice, and the concurrent disqualification of intuitive knowledge in medical decision making, see Deborah Gordon, "Clinical Science and Clinical Expertise: Changing Boundaries Between Art and Science in Medicine," in *Biomedicine Examined*, edited by Margaret Lock and Deborah Gordon (Boston: Kluwer Academic Publishers, 1988).

11. Susan Bell, "Becoming a Political Woman: The Reconstruction and Interpretation of Experience through Stories," in *Gender and Discourse: The Power of Talk*, edited by Alexandra Dundas Todd and Sue Fisher (Norwood: Ablex Publishing Corp., 1988), 97–123.

12. Ibid., 120.

13. Ibid., 116.

14. Ibid., 99.

15. Ibid., 116.

16. Eve chose to trust her conviction that her implants were causing her health problems and eventually did have her breast implants removed. I learned this information during my second interview with her in 1997.

17. These women were Ann, Carmen, Tracy, Mary, Maureen, and Kate.

18. Ann and Tracy were the only two women out of this group of six who were fearful about the possible long-term health effects of their breast implants. Tracy had begun to network with national organizations for implant recipients, and Ann talked to me about starting her own support group.

19. Although most of the evidence in my analysis was derived from women's accounts of their own experiences, occasionally I relied on women's speculations about other women they had come in contact with who had received breast implants. In particular, support group leaders provided me with a wealth of information about the women in their groups.

20. A woman's willingness and ability to find support was not necessarily dependent on her socioeconomic status. Indeed, I spoke with several women whose total household incomes were extremely low and whose educational history was minimal but who nevertheless were actively involved in support groups for women with breast implants. Since my sample consisted of mostly white, American-born women, I cannot make the same type of conclusion with regard to race and ethnicity.

21. As indicated in the previous chapter, Barbara is much more willing to accept the possibility that her implants are causing her health problems today than she was during our initial interview two and a half years ago. She explained that her health has deteriorated to such an extent that she feels she has little choice now but to accept the possibility that her implants are to blame for her worsening symptoms.

Chapter Eight

1. Kathy Davis, *Reshaping the Female Body: The Dilemma of Cosmetic Surgery* (New York: Routledge, 1995).

2. Ibid., 149.

3. Ibid., 143.

4. Ibid., 143.

5. Ibid., 137.

6. Ibid., 151.

7. Ibid., 11.

8. Ibid., 153.

9. Ibid.

10. See Barbara's story in Chapter 7 in the section headed "Class and Ethnic Barriers to Finding Support."

11. Davis, *Reshaping the Female Body*, 151.

12. Ibid., 157.

13. Ann Bookman and Sandra Morgen, *Women and the Politics of Empowerment* (Philadelphia: Temple University Press, 1988), 4.

14. However, in Chapter 4, I also explain that half of the women I interviewed were initially dissatisfied with the outcomes of their surgeries. Hoping that larger breasts would improve their sexual and social lives, these women felt more objectified and disconnected from their true identities following their surgeries. Having implants made them feel like "fakes" and "frauds." They explained that they were ashamed that they had given in to cultural ideals of femininity and female bodily appearance, and they chose to keep their implants a secret from friends, potential lovers, and family members.

15. Also see Davis, *Reshaping the Female Body.*

16. This is true especially in cases of implant rupture. If silicone has migrated into surrounding breast tissue, frequently a mastectomy must be performed.

17. A few women also explained that insurance companies refused to reimburse them for implant removal. Also see Joan Rigdon, "Women Find It Difficult to Get Breast Implants Removed," *Wall Street Journal,* Mar. 20, 1992. Third-party payers are willing to reimburse only for surgeries deemed by physicians to be "medically necessary." This policy presented a problem for many of the women I interviewed whose plastic surgeons were unwilling to acknowledge the possibility that breast implants are related to certain symptoms and diseases.

18. See Chapter 3.

19. The factors that played into women's decisions to have breast implants for reconstructive purposes following mastectomies are discussed in Chapter 3.

20. See Arlene Skolnick and Jerome Skolnick, *Family in Transition: Rethinking Marriage, Sexuality, Child Rearing, and Family Organization,* 8th ed. (New York: HarperCollins, 1994).

21. Similarly, Parnel Wickham-Searl explored the nature of authority and the emergence of expertise among mothers of children with disabilities, finding that women's stories "revealed a changing dynamic in their lives that shifted the focus of authority from those presumed to be knowledgeable on account of their professional status, to themselves, women vested with the authority of raising children who were disabled"; see "Mothers of Children with Disabilities and the Construction of Expertise," *Research in Sociology of Health Care* 11 (1994): 180.

22. Peter Conrad similarly argues that what is interpreted by physicians as "noncompliance" may be interpreted by patients as a move to take more responsibility over their lives; see Peter Conrad, "The Noncompliant Patient in Search for Autonomy," *Hastings Center Report* 17 (1987): 15–17.

23. Also see Norman Fineman, "The Social Construction of Noncompliance: A Study of Health Care and Social Service Providers in Everyday Practice," *Sociology of Health and Illness* 13 (1991): 354–74.

24. James Trostle, "Medical Compliance as an Ideology," *Social Science and Medicine* 27 (1988): 1299.

Bibliography

American Society of Plastic and Reconstructive Surgeons. 1982. *Position Statement*.
———. 1992. *Position Statement*.
Angell, Marcia. 1992. "Breast Implants—Protection or Paternalism?" Editorial. *New England Journal of Medicine* 326: 1695–98.
———. 1996. *Science on Trial: The Clash of Medical Evidence and the Law in the Breast Implant Case*. New York: W. W. Norton.
Apfel, Roberta, and Susan Fisher. 1984. *To Do No Harm: DES and the Dilemmas of Modern Medicine*. New Haven: Yale University Press.
Baker, Nancy C. 1984. *The Beauty Trap: Exploring Woman's Greatest Obsession*. New York: Franklin Watts.
Barker-Benfield, Graham John. 1976. *The Horrors of the Half-Known Life: Male Attitudes toward Women and Sexuality in 19th Century America*. New York: Harper & Row.
Bell, Susan. 1986. "A New Model of Medical Technology Development: A Case Study of DES." *Research in the Sociology of Health Care* 4: 1–32.
———. 1987. "Changing Ideas: The Medicalization of Menopause." *Social Science and Medicine* 24: 535–42.
———. 1988. "Becoming a Political Woman: The Reconstruction and Interpretation of Experience through Stories." In *Gender and Discourse: The Power of Talk*, edited by Alexandra Dundas Todd and Sue Fisher. Norwood: Ablex Publishing.
———. 1989. "Technology in Medicine: Development, Diffusion, and Health Policy." In *Handbook of Medical Sociology*, edited by Howard Freeman and Sol Levine. Englewood Cliffs, N.J.: Prentice Hall.
———. 1995. "Gendered Medical Science: Producing a Drug for Women." *Feminist Studies* 21: 469–500.
———. 1997. "Technology Assessment, Outcome Data and Social Context: The Case of Hormone Therapy." In *Getting Doctors to Listen*, edited by P. Boyle. Washington, D.C.: Georgetown University Press.
Berkel, Hans, Dale Birdsell, and Heather Jenkins. 1992. "Breast Augmentation: A Risk Factor for Breast Cancer?" *New England Journal of Medicine* 326: 1649–53.
Bonavoglia, Angela. 1996. "Alternatives: Know the Risks." *Ms.* 6: 58.

213

Bookman, Ann, and Sandra Morgen. 1988. *Women and the Politics of Empowerment.* Philadelphia: Temple University Press.

Bordo, Susan. 1993. *Unbearable Weight: Feminism, Western Culture, and the Body.* Berkeley and Los Angeles: University of California Press.

Bridges, Alan, Carol Conley, Grace Wang, David Burns, and Frank Vasey. 1993. "A Clinical Immunological Evaluation of Women with Silicone Breast Implants and Symptoms of Rheumatic Disease." *Annals of Internal Medicine* 118: 929–36.

Brody, G. S., D. P. Conway, D. M. Deapen, J. C. Fisher, M. C. Hochberg, E. C. Leroy, T. A. Medsger Jr., M. C. Robson, A. R. Shons, and M. H. Weisman. 1992. "Consensus Statement on the Relationship of Breast Implant to Connective-Tissue Disorders." *Plastic and Reconstructive Surgery* 90: 1102–5.

Brown, Phil. 1992. "Popular Epidemiology and Toxic Waste Contamination: Lay and Professional Ways of Knowing." *Journal of Health and Social Behavior* 33: 267–81.

Brown, Phil, and Edwin Mikkelsen. 1990. *No Safe Place: Toxic Waste, Leukemia, and Community Action.* Berkeley: University of California Press.

Brownmiller, Susan. 1984. *Femininity.* New York: Linden Press / Simon and Schuster.

Bruning, Nancy. 1995. *Breast Implants: Everything You Need to Know.* 2d ed. Alameda, Calif.: Hunter House.

Burton, Thomas. 1992. "How Industrial Foam Came to Be Employed in Breast Implants." *Wall Street Journal,* Mar. 25.

———. 1993. "Breast Implants Raise More Safety Issues." *Wall Street Journal,* Feb. 4.

———. 1997. "Frequency of Reoperations for Women with Breast Implants Put at Nearly Twenty-five Percent." *Wall Street Journal,* Mar. 6.

Byrne, John. 1996. *Informed Consent: A Story of Personal Tragedy and Corporate Betrayal.* New York: McGraw-Hill.

Chapkis, Wendy. 1986. *Beauty Secrets: Women and the Politics of Appearance.* Boston: South End Press.

Chrisler, Joan, and Karen Levy. 1990. "The Media Construct of a Menstrual Monster." *Women and Health* 16: 89–104.

Clarke, Adele. 1990. "Women's Health: Life-Cycle Issues." In *Women, Health, and Medicine in America,* edited by Rima Apple. New York: Garland Publishing.

Cohen, S. B., and R. J. Rohrich. 1994. "Evaluation of the Patient with Silicone Breast Implants and Rheumatic Complaints." *Plastic and Reconstructive Surgery* 94: 120–25.

Conrad, Peter. 1987. "The Noncompliant Patient in Search for Autonomy." *Hastings Center Report* 17: 15–17.

———. 1992. "Medicalization and Social Control." *Annual Review of Sociology* 18: 209–32.

Conway, Herbert, and Dicran Goulian. 1963. "Experience with an Injectable Silastic RTV as a Subcutaneous Prosthetic Material." *Plastic and Reconstructive Surgery* 32: 294–302.

Cook, Linda, Janet R. Daling, Linda F. Voigt, M. Patricia DeHart, Kathleen E. Malone, Janet L. Stanford, Noel S. Weiss, Louise A. Brinton, Marilie D. Gammon, and Donna Brogan. 1997. "Characteristics of Women With and Without Breast Augmentation." *Journal of the American Medical Association* 277: 1612–17.

Cook, Ralph, Robert Delongchamp, Maryann Woodbury, Laura Perkins, and Myron Harrison. 1995. "The Prevalence of Women with Breast Implants in the United States—1989." *Journal of Clinical Epidemiology* 48: 519–25.

Davis, Kathy. 1991. "Remaking the She-Devil: A Critical Look at Feminist Approaches to Beauty." *Hypatia* 6: 23.

———. 1993. "Cultural Dopes and She-Devils: Cosmetic Surgery as Ideological Dilemma." In *Negotiating at the Margins: The Gendered Discourses of Power and Resistance*, edited by Kathy Davis and Sue Fisher. New Brunswick, N.J.: Rutgers University Press.

———. 1995. *Reshaping the Female Body: The Dilemma of Cosmetic Surgery*. New York: Routledge.

Deapen D. M., M. C. Pike, J. T. Casagrande, and G. S. Brody. 1986. "The Relationship between Breast Cancer and Augmentation Mammaplasty: An Epidemiological Study." *Plastic and Reconstructive Surgery* 77: 361–67.

Deapen, Dennis, and Garry Brody. 1995. "Augmentation Mammaplasty and Breast Cancer: A Five Year Update of the Los Angeles Study." *Journal of Clinical Epidemiology* 48: 551–56.

Dow Brochure. 1976. "Facts You Should Know About Your New Look."

Dow Document. 1976. Jan. 15.

———. 1975. May 16.

Duffy, M. J., and J. E. Woods. 1994. "Health Risks of Failed Silicone Gel Breast Implants." *Plastic and Reconstructive Surgery* 94: 295–99.

Dugowson, C., J. Daling, T. Koepsell, L. Voight, and J. Nelson. 1992. "Silicone Breast Implants and Risk for Rheumatoid Arthritis." *Arthritis and Rheumatism* 35: S66.

Dull, Diana, and Candace West. 1991. "Accounting for Cosmetic Surgery: The Accomplishment of Gender." *Social Problems* 38: 54–95.

Edgerton, M. T., and A. R. McClary. 1958. "Augmentation Mammaplasty: Psychiatric Implications and Surgical Indications." *Plastic and Reconstructive Surgery* 21: 279–305.

Edgerton, M.T., E. Meyer, and W.E. Jacobson. 1961. "Augmentation Mammaplasty: Further Surgical and Psychiatric Evaluation." *Plastic and Reconstructive Surgery* 27: 279–302.

Ehrenreich, Barbara, and Deirdre English. 1989. *For Her Own Good: 150 Years of the Experts' Advice to Women*. New York: Doubleday.

Endo, L. P., N. L. Edwards, S. Longley, L. C. Corman, R. S. Panush. 1987. "Silicone and Rheumatic Diseases." *Seminars in Arthritis and Rheumatism* 17: 112–18.

Engel, Arnold, Steven Lamm, and Sheghan Lai. 1995. "Human Breast Sarcoma and Human Breast Implantation." *Journal of Clinical Epidemiology* 48: 539–44.

Fausto-Sterling, Anne. 1992. *Myths of Gender: Biological Theories about Women and Men*. New York: Basic Books.

Federal Register. 1988. 53: 23,856–77.

———. 1993. 58: 3438–39.

Fineman, Norman. 1991. "The Social Construction of Noncompliance: A Study of Health Care and Social Service Providers in Everyday Practice." *Sociology of Health and Illness* 13: 354–74.

Finley, Lucinda. 1994. Statement presented before the Subcommittee on Courts and Administrative Practice of the Committee on the Judiciary of the United States Senate on S.687—The Product Liability Fairness Act, 103d Congress, 2d Session.

Fisher, Jack. 1992. "The Silicone Controversy—When Will Science Prevail?" *New England Journal of Medicine* 326: 196–98.

Fisher, Sue. 1983. "Doctor Talk/Patient Talk: How Treatment Decisions are Negotiated in Doctor-Patient Communication." In *The Social Organization of Medicine*, edited by Sue Fisher and Alexandra Dundas Todd. Washington, D.C.: Center for Applied Linguistics.

———. 1986. *In the Patient's Best Interest: Women and the Politics of Medical Decisions.* New Brunswick, N.J.: Rutgers University Press.

Foucault, Michel. 1979. *Discipline and Punishment.* New York: Vintage Books.

Frank, Henry. 1987. "Violence Against Women: The Pharmaceutical Industry." *Free Inquiry in Creative Sociology* 15: 199–205.

Freedman, Rita. 1986. *Beauty Bound.* Lexington, Mass.: Lexington Books.

Gabriel, Sherine, Michael O'Fallon, C. Mary Beard, Leonard Kurland, John Woods, and L. Joseph Melton III. 1995. "Trends in the Utilization of Silicone Breast Implants, 1964–1991, and Methodology for a Population-Based Study of Outcomes." *Journal of Clinical Epidemiology* 48: 527–37.

Gabriel, Sherine, Michael O'Fallon, Leonard Kurland, Mary Beard, John Woods, and Joseph Melton. 1994. "Risk of Connective Tissue Disease and Other Disorders after Breast Implantation." *New England Journal of Medicine* 330: 1697–1702.

Gabriel, Sherine, John Woods, Michael O'Fallon, Mary Beard, Leonard Kurland, and Joseph Melton III. 1997. "Complications Leading to Surgery after Breast Implantation." *New England Journal of Medicine* 336: 677–82.

Garfinkle, Harold, and Egon Bittner. 1967. "'Good' Organizational Reasons for 'Bad' Clinical Records." In *Studies in Ethnomethodology*, edited by Harold Garfinkle. Englewood Cliffs, N.J.: Prentice Hall.186–207.

Garland, Anne Witte. 1988. *Women Activists: Challenging the Abuse of Power.* New York: Feminist Press at the City University of New York.

Gelijns, Annetine C., and Alan Moskowitz. 1996. "Derelictions." *Science* 273: 917.

Gilbert, Nigel, and Christian Heath. 1986. "Text, Competence and Logic: An Exercise." *Qualitative Sociology* 9: 215–36.

Giltay, E., H. Moens, A. Riley, and R. Tan. 1994. "Silicone Breast Prostheses and Rheumatic Symptoms: A Retrospective Follow-up Study." *Annals of Rheumatic Disorders* 53: 194–96.

Goldman, John, Jesse Greenblatt, Ron Joines, Leslie White, Bruce Aylward, and Steven Lamm. 1995. "Breast Implants, Rheumatoid Arthritis, and Connective Tissue Disease in a Clinical Practice." *Journal of Clinical Epidemiology* 48: 571–82.

Good, Byron, and Mary-Jo Delvecchio Good. 1993. "'Learning Medicine': The Construction of Knowledge at Harvard Medical School." In *Knowledge, Power and Practice*, edited by Shirley Lindenbaum and Margaret Lock. Berkeley: University of California Press.

Gordon, Deborah. 1988. "Clinical Science and Clinical Expertise: Changing Boundaries Between Art and Science in Medicine." In *Biomedicine Examined*, edited by Margaret Lock and Deborah Gordon. Boston: Kluwer Academic Publishers.

————. 1988. "Tenacious Assumptions in Western Medicine." In *Biomedicine Examined*, edited by Margaret Lock and Deborah Gordon. Boston: Kluwer Academic Publishers.

Graham, Judith. 1997. "Increased Offer on Implants Assailed: Dow Corning Would Pay Out $2.4 Billion in Settlement." *Chicago Tribune*, Aug. 26.

Guidon, R., M. Therrien, C. Rolland, M. King, J. L. Grandmaison, S. Kaliaguine, P. Blais, H. Pakdel, and C. Roy. 1992. "The Polyurethane Foam Covering the Meme Breast Prosthesis: A Biomedical Breakthrough or a Biomaterial Tar baby?" *Annals of Plastic Surgery* 28: 342–53.

Guillemin, Jeanne. 1994. "Experiment and Illusion in Reproductive Medicine." *Human Nature* 5: 1–22.

Haney, Daniel. 1994. "Medical Editor's Role as Expert Paid by Lawyers Is Scrutinized." *Boston Globe*, Dec. 12.

Hay, G. G. 1970. "Psychiatric Aspects of Cosmetic Nasal Operations." *British Journal of Psychiatry* 116: 85–97.

Hayes, H., M. S. Vandergrift, and W. C. Diner. 1988. "Mammography and Breast Implants." *Plastic and Reconstructive Surgery* 82: 1–6.

Health Facts, "Silicone Breast Implants: Serious Problems are Virtually Guaranteed." New York: Center for Medical Consumers Inc., Dec. 1989, 4–6.

Hennekens, Charles, I-Min Lee, Nancy Cook, Patricia Herbert, Elizabeth Karlson, Fran LaMotte, JoAnn Manson, and Julie Buring. 1996. "Self-Reported Breast Implants and Connective Tissue Diseases in Female Health Professionals: A Retrospective Cohort Study." *Journal of the American Medical Association* 275: 616–21.

Hidalgo, David. 1990. "Breast Reconstruction." In *Women Talk about Breast Surgery: From Diagnosis to Recovery*, edited by Amy Gross and Dee Ito. New York: Harper Perennial.

Hill, G., and A. G. Silver. 1950. "Psychodynamic and Aesthetic Modifications for Plastic Surgery." *Psychosomatic Medicine* 12: 345.

Hilts, Philip J. 1992. "Silicone: Friend or Foe? Strange History of Silicone Held Many Warning Signs." *New York Times*, Jan. 18.

————. 1992. "Company to Release Data Questioning Implant Safety." *New York Times*, Jan. 23.

Hochberg, Marc, Robyn Miller, and Fredrick Wigley. 1995. "Frequency of Augmentation Mammoplasty in Patients with Systemic Sclerosis: Data from the Johns Hopkins–University of Maryland Scleroderma Center." *Journal of Clinical Epidemiology* 48: 565–69.

Human Resources and Intergovernmental Relations Subcommittee of the Committee on Governmental Operations. 1993. *The FDA's Regulation of Silicone Breast Implants.* Washington, D.C.: Government Printing Office.

Jacobson, W. E., M. T. Edgerton, E. Meyer, A. Canter, and R. Slaughter. 1960. "Psychiatric Evaluation of Male Patients Seeking Cosmetic Surgery." *Plastic and Reconstructive Surgery* 26: 356.

Jacobus, Mary, Evelyn Fox Keller, and Sally Shuttleworth. 1990. *Body/Politics: Women and the Discourses of Science*. New York: Routledge.

Jaggar, Alison. 1983. *Feminist Politics and Human Nature*. Sussex, Eng.: Harvester Press, Ltd.

Jaggar, Alison, and Susan Bordo, eds. 1989. *Gender/Body/Knowledge*. New Brunswick, N.J.: Rutgers University Press.

Kaiser, W., G. Biesenbach, U. Stuby, P. Grafinger, J. Zazgornik. 1990. "Human Adjuvant Disease: Remission of Silicone Induces Autoimmune Disease after Explantation of Breast Augmentation." *Annals of Rheumatic Disorders* 49: 937–38.

Kaw, Eugena. 1993. "Medicalization of Racial Features: Asian American Women and Cosmetic Surgery." *Medical Anthropology Quarterly* 7: 74–89.

Keithley-Johnston, Kathy. 1997. "Victims of Faulty Implants Fight Enemies Within, Without." *Columbia Daily Tribune*, Mar. 11.

Keller, Evelyn Fox. 1992. *Secrets of Life and Death: Essays on Language, Gender and Science*. New York: Routledge.

Kessler, David A. 1992. "The Basis of the FDA's Decision on Breast Implants." *New England Journal of Medicine* 326: 1713–15.

Kleinman, Arthur. 1988. *The Illness Narratives: Suffering, Healing and the Human Condition*. New York: Basic Books.

Kolata, Gina. 1994. "3 Breast Implant Makers Agree to Pay $3.7 Billion." *New York Times*, Feb. 20.

———. 1995. "Implant Lawsuits Create a Medical Rush to Cash In." *New York Times*, Sept. 9.

———. 1995. "Proof of Breast Implant Peril Is Lacking, Rheumatologists Say." *New York Times*, Oct. 26. 1995.

———. 1996. "Study Cites Small Risks for Women From Breast Implants." *New York Times*, Feb. 28.

———. 1997. "Dow Corning Seeks to Settle Implant Case." *New York Times*, Aug. 26.

Kong, Dolores. 1996. "Breast Implant Study Finds Some Risk." *Boston Globe*, Feb. 28.

Kumagai, Yauo, Yuichi Shiokawa, Thomas Medsger Jr., and Gerald Rodnan. 1984. "Clinical Spectrum of Connective Tissue Disease after Cosmetic Surgery." *Arthritis and Rheumatism* 27: 1–12.

La Leche League International. 1992. *Nursing with Breast Implants*.

Lappé, Marc. 1991. *Chemical Deception: The Toxic Threat to Health and the Environment*. San Francisco: Sierra Club Books.

———. 1993. "Silicone Reactive Disorder: A New Autoimmune Disease Caused by Immunostimulation and Superantigens." *Medical Hypothesis* 41: 348–52.

———. 1994. *Evolutionary Medicine: Rethinking the Origins of Disease*. San Francisco: Sierra Club Books.

Leibman, Jill A., Marjorie Kossoff, and Beth D. Kruse. 1992. "Intraductal Extension of Silicone from a Ruptured Breast Implant." *Plastic and Reconstructive Surgery* 89: 546–47.

Levine, J. J., and N. T. Ilowite. 1994. "Scleroderma-like Esophageal Disease in Children Breast-fed by Mothers with Silicone Breast Implants." *Journal of the American Medical Association* 271: 213–16.

Lloyd, Marilyn. 1995. "The Real Tragedy Behind Silicone Breast Implants." *Chicago Tribune*, Nov. 9.

Lorde, Audre. 1980. *The Cancer Journals*. San Francisco: Spinsters Ink.

McCarthy, E. Jane, Ruth Merkatz, and Grant Bagley. 1993. "A Descriptive Analysis of Physical Complaints from Women with Silicone Breast Implants." *Journal of Women's Health* 2: 111–15.

Martin, Emily. 1992. *The Woman in the Body: A Cultural Analysis of Reproduction*. 2d ed. Boston: Beacon Press.

———. 1994. *Flexible Bodies: Tracking Immunity in American Culture—From the Days of Polio to the Age of AIDS*. Boston: Beacon Press.

Merkatz, Ruth, Grant Bagley, and Jane McCarthy. 1993. "A Qualitative Analysis of Self-Reported Experiences among Women Encountering Difficulties with Silicone Breast Implants." *Journal of Women's Health* 2: 105–15.

Meyerowitz, Beth, Shelly Chaiken, and Laura Clark. 1988. "Sexual Roles and Culture: Social and Personal Reactions to Breast Cancer." In *Women with Disabilities: Essays in Psychology, Culture and Politics*, edited by Michelle Fine and Adrienne Asch. Philadelphia: Temple University Press.

Millman, Marcia. 1980. *Such a Pretty Face: Being Fat in America*. New York: Norton.

Mills, C. Wright. 1959. *The Sociological Imagination*. New York: Oxford University Press.

Mintz, Morton. 1985. *At Any Cost: Corporate Greed, Women and the Dalkon Shield*. New York: Pantheon Books.

Mishler, Elliot. 1981. "Critical Perspectives on the Biomedical Model." In *Social Contexts of Health, Illness, and Patient Care*, edited by Elliot Mishler, Lorna Amara Singham, Stuart T. Hauser, Ramsay Liem, Samuel Osherson, and Nancy E. Waxler. Cambridge: Cambridge University Press.

———. 1984. *The Discourse of Medicine: Dialectics of Medical Interviews*. Norwood: Ablex Publishing.

Morgan, Robert, and Maryellen Elcock. 1995. "Artificial Implants and Soft Tissue Sarcomas." *Journal of Clinical Epidemiology* 48: 545–49.

Naim, J. O., R. J. Lanzafame, J. C. Van Oss. 1993. "The Adjuvant Effect of Silicone-Gel on Antibody Formation in Rats." *Immunological Investigations* 22: 151–61.

Oakley, Ann 1981. "Interviewing Women: A Contradiction in Terms." In *Doing Feminist Research*, edited by Helen Roberts. Boston: Routledge and Kegan Paul.

Okano, Y., M. Nishikai, and A. Sato. 1984. "Scleroderma, Primary Biliary Cirrhosis, and Sjögren's Syndrome after Breast Augmentation with Silicone Injection: A Case Report of Possible Adjuvant Disease." *Annals of Rheumatic Disorders* 43: 520–22.

Oppenheimer, B. S., E. T. Oppenheimer, and A. P. Stout. 1952. "Sarcomas Induced in Rodents by Embedding Various Plastic Films." *Proceedings of the Society for Experimental Biology and Medicine* 79: 366.

Paletta C., F. X. Paletta Jr., and F. X. Paletta Sr. 1992. "Squamous Cell Carcinoma Following Breast Augmentation." *Annals of Plastic Surgery* 29: 425–29.

Peters, W., E. Keystone, K. Snow, L. Rubin, D. Smith. 1994. "Is There a Relationship between Autoantibodies and Silicone-gel Implants?" *Annals of Plastic Surgery* 21: 5–7.

Peters, Walter, and Dennis Smith. 1981. "Ivalon Sponge Prostheses: Evaluation of 19 Years after Implantation." *Plastic and Reconstructive Surgery* 67: 514–18.

Petit, J. Y., M. G. Lee, H. Mouriesse, M. Rietjens, P. Gill, G. Contesso, and A. Lehmann. 1994. "Can Reconstruction with Gel-Filled Silicone Implants Increase the Risk of Death and Second Primary Cancer in Patients Treated by Mastectomy for Breast Cancer?" *Plastic and Reconstructive Surgery* 94: 115–19.

Pollock, Harlan. 1993. "Breast Capsular Contracture: A Retrospective Study of Textured versus Smooth Silicone Breast Implants." *Plastic and Reconstructive Surgery* 91: 404–7.

Potter, M., S. Morrison, F. Wiener, K. X. Zhang, and F. Miller. 1994. "Induction of Plasmacytomas with Silicone Gel in Genetically Susceptible Strains of Mice." *Journal of the National Cancer Institute* 86: 1058–65.

Project Impact. 1995. *Impact!* (Newsletter), Apr.

Reuters, 1993. "Dow Corning Cites Subpoena for Falsified Implant Data." *Boston Globe*, Feb. 18.

Riessman, Catherine Kohler. 1983. "Women and Medicalization: A New Perspective." *Social Policy* 14: 3–18.

———. 1993. *Narrative Analysis*. Newbury Park, Calif.: Sage Publications.

Rigdon, Joan E. 1992. "Women Find It Difficult to Get Breast Implants Removed." *Wall Street Journal*, Mar. 20.

———. 1993. "Saline Implants Now Seem to Carry Health Hazards as Well." *Wall Street Journal*, Feb. 4.

Rittenhouse, Amanda. 1991. "The Emergence of Premenstrual Syndrome as a Social Problem." *Social Problems* 38: 412–25.

Rosenberg, Charles. 1996. "The Silicone Papers." Review of *Science on Trial: The Clash of Medical Evidence and the Law in the Breast Implant Case*, by Marcia Angell. *New York Times* (book review section), July 14.

Rothman, Barbara Katz. 1991. *In Labor: Women and Power in the Birthplace*. New York: W. W. Norton.

Ruzek, Sheryl. 1986. "Feminist Visions of Health: An International Perspective." In *What Is Feminism?* edited by Ann Oakley and Juliet Mitchell. New York: Pantheon Books.

Salmon, Sydney, and Robert Kyle. 1994. "Silicone Gels, Induction of Plasma Cell Tumors, and Genetic Susceptibility in Mice: A Call for Epidemiological Investigation of Women with Silicone Breast Implants." *Journal of the National Cancer Institute* 86: 1040–41.

Sanchez-Guerro, J., P. H. Schur, and M. H. Liang. 1994. "Silicone Breast Implants and Rheumatic Disease." *Arthritis and Rheumatism* 37: 158–68.

Sandelowski, Margarete. 1981. *Women, Health and Choice*. Englewood Cliffs, N.J.: Prentice Hall Inc.

Schneider, Joseph, and Peter Conrad. 1980. "In the Closet with Illness: Epilepsy, Stigma Potential and Information Control." *Social Problems* 28: 32–44.

Schwartz, A. W., and J. B. Erich. 1960. "Experimental Study of Polyvinyl-formula (Ivalon) Sponge as a Substitute for Tissue." *Plastic and Reconstructive Surgery* 25: 1.

Schwartz, Miriam A. 1984. "A Sociological Reinterpretation of the Controversy over 'Unnecessary Surgery.'" *Research in the Sociology of Health Care* 3: 169–200.

Seaman, Barbara, and Seaman Gideon. 1977. *Women and the Crisis of Sex Hormones.* New York: Rawson Associates Publishers.

Shmerling, Robert, and Matthew Liang. 1993. "Laboratory Evaluation of Rheumatic Diseases." In *Primer on the Rheumatic Diseases.* Atlanta: The Arthritis Foundation.

Shoaib, B. O., B. M. Patten, and D. S. Caulkin. 1994. "Adjuvant Breast Disease: An Evaluation of 100 Symptomatic Women with Breast Implants or Silicone Fluid Injections." *Keio Journal of Medicine* 43: 79–87.

Showalter, Elaine. 1981. "Victorian Women and Insanity." In *Madhouses, Mad-Doctors, and Madmen: The Social History of Psychiatry in the Victorian Era*, edited by Andrew Scull. Philadelphia: University of Pennsylvania Press.

Silver, R. M., E. E. Sahn, A. J. Allen, S. Sahn, W. Greene, J. C. Maize, and P. D. Garen. 1993. "Demonstration of Silicon in Sites of Connective-Tissue Disease in Patients with Silicone Gel Breast Implants." *Archives of Dermatology* 129: 63–68.

Silverman, B. G., S. L. Brown, R. A. Bright, R. G. Kaczmarek, J. B. Arrowsmith-Lowe, and D. A. Kessler. 1996. "Reported Complications of Silicone Gel Breast Implants: An Epidemiological Review." *Annals of Internal Medicine* 124: 744–56.

Skolnick, Arlene, and Jerome Skolnick. 1994. *Family in Transition: Rethinking Marriage, Sexuality, Child Rearing and Family Organization.* 8th ed. New York: HarperCollins.

Spiera, H. 1988. "Scleroderma after Silicone Augmentation Mammoplasty." *Journal of the American Medical Association* 260: 236–38.

Spierra, R. F., A. Gibofsky, and H. Spiera. 1994. "Silicone Gel-Filled Breast Implants and Connective Tissue Disease: An Overview." *Journal of Rheumatology* 21: 239–45.

Spitzack, Carole. 1990. *Confessing Excess: Women and the Politics of Body Reduction.* Albany: State University of New York Press.

Starr, Paul. 1982. *The Social Transformation of American Medicine.* New York: Basic Books.

Tenenbaum, Scott, Janet Rice, Luis Espinoza, Marta Cuéllar, Douglas Plymae, Davis Sander, Linda Williamson, Allyson Haislip, Oscar Gluck, John Tesser, Less Nogy, Kathleen Stribrny, Julie Bevan, and Robert Garry. 1997. "Use of Anti-Polymer Assay in Recipients of Silicone Breast Implants." *Lancet* 349: 449–54.

Terry, Mary Beth, Mary Louise Skovron, Samantha Garbers, Elizabeth Sonnen-schein, and Paolo Toniolo. 1995. "The Estimated Frequency of Cosmetic Breast Augmentation among US Women, 1963 through 1988." *American Journal of Public Health* 85: 1122–24.

Teuber, S. S., and M. E. Gershwin. 1994. "Autoantibodies and Clinical Rheumatic Complaints in Two Children of Women with Silicone Gel Breast Implants." *International Archives of Allergy and Immunology* 103: 105–8.

Todd, Alexandra Dundas. 1983. "Women's Bodies as Diseased and Deviant." *Research in Law, Deviance, and Social Control* 5: 83–95.

———. 1984. "The Prescription of Contraception: Negotiations Between Doctors and Patients." *Discourse Processes* 7: 171–200.

———. 1989. *Intimate Adversaries: Cultural Conflict Between Doctors and Women Patients*. Philadelphia: University of Pennsylvania Press.

———. 1994. *Double Vision: An East-West Collaboration for Coping with Cancer*. Hanover, N.H.: University Press of New England.

Travis, Cheryl Brown. 1985. "Medical Decision Making and Elective Surgery: The Case of Hysterectomy." *Risk Analysis* 5: 241–51.

Trostle, James. 1988. "Medical Compliance as an Ideology." *Social Science and Medicine* 27: 1299–1308.

U.S. Department of Health and Human Services. 1993. *HHS News* Jan. 5.

Updegraff, Howard, and Karl Menninger. 1934. "Some Psychoanalytic Aspects of Plastic Surgery." *American Journal of Surgery* 25: 554–58.

Uretsky, B. F., J. J. O'Brien, E. H. Courtiss, et al. 1979. "Augmentation Mammoplasty Associated with a Severe Systemic Illness." *Annals of Plastic Surgery* 3: 445–47.

Vasey, Frank, and Josh Feldstein. 1993. *The Silicone Breast Implant Controversy: What Women Need to Know*. Freedom, Calif.: Crossing Press.

Vaughan, Mary. 1997. "A Head-on Collision with 'Junk Science.'" *Chicago Tribune*, Apr. 3.

Waitzkin, Howard. 1983. *The Second Sickness: Contradictions of Capitalist Health Care*. New York: Free Press.

———. 1989. "A Critical Theory of Medical Discourse: Ideology, Social Control, and the Processing of Social Context in Medical Encounters." *Journal of Health and Social Behavior* 30: 220–39.

Wallen, J. 1979. "Physician Stereotypes about Female Health and Illness." *Women and Health* 4: 135–46.

Wear, Delese. 1993. "'Your Breasts/Sliced Off': Literary Images of Breast Cancer." *Women and Health* 20: 81–100.

Wells, K. E., C. W. Cruse, J. L. Baker, S. M. Daniel, R. A. Stern, C. Newman, M. J. Seleznick, F. B. Vasey, S. Brozana, and S. E. Albers. 1994. "The Health Status of Women Following Cosmetic Surgery." *Plastic and Reconstructive Surgery* 93: 907–12.

West, Candace. 1993. "Reconceptualizing Gender in Physician-Patient Relationships." *Social Science and Medicine* 36: 57–66.

"Why Judges Must Fight Bad Science: Big Settlement in Silicone Implant Cases Reveals Problem." 1995. Editorial. *Los Angeles Times*, June 28.

Wickham-Searl, Parnel. 1994. "Mothers of Children with Disabilities and the Construction of Expertise." *Research in Sociology of Health Care* 11: 175–87.

Williams, Gareth. 1984. "The Genesis of Chronic Illness: Narrative Reconstruction." *Sociology of Health and Illness* 6: 176–200.

Wronski, Richard. 1995. "Rheumatologists See No Danger in Silicone Devices." *Chicago Tribune*, Oct. 26.

Young, Iris. 1990. *Throwing Like a Girl and Other Essays in Feminist Philosophy and Social Theory*. Bloomington: Indiana University Press.

Zola, Irving. 1991. "Bringing Our Bodies and Ourselves Back In: Reflections on a Past, Present, and Future Medical Sociology." *Journal of Health and Social Behavior* 32: 1–16.

Index

Aesthech Corporation, 31
American Medical Association, 97, 109–10
American Society of Plastic and Reconstructive Surgeons, 6, 7, 12, 37, 40, 106, 109; definition of cosmetic surgery, 61
Angell, Marcia, 13–14, 38, 139–40, 143
autoimmune disease: associated with breast implants, 3, 38, 39, 111, 119, 123, 128, 130, 141, 149

Bell, Susan, 97, 126, 157
Blizzard, Ed, 36–37
Bookman, Ann, 173
Bordo, Susan, 44–46, 47, 98
Braley, Silas, 28
breast cancer, 38; reconstructive surgery following, 62–69. *See also* mastectomy
breast-feeding: effect of implants on, 40–41, 111–12
breast implants, saline, 30, 106–7, 122–23
breast implants, silicone: anger as reaction following, 74–75, 117, 128–29, 133, 146; autoimmune disease associated with, 3, 38, 39, 111, 119, 123, 128, 130, 141, 149; before-and-after photos of, 70–71, 113; and breast-feeding, 40–41, 111–12; and cancer risk, 39–40; complications associated with, 21, 29, 38–39, 79–80, 95–96, 185–86; and connective-tissue disease, 39; cultural influences on decision, 71–73, 89–90, 96–100, 112–14, 117–18, 189; decision to seek, 42–69, 71–72, 179; development of, 28–29; dichotomy between patients' and physicians' view of, 147–48, 165–66, 185–89; as empowering experi-

ence, 78, 89, 98, 171, 172, 173; expectations versus reality of, 70–90; gel-filled, 29–30, 32–37; government regulation of, 2, 6, 14, 21, 29, 31–32, 34–35, 107–10, 140; hardening of, 120, 126; historical background, 20–41; impact of, on relationships, 180–84; impact of, on sexuality, 16; informed consent forms for, 109–10; insurance coverage of, 9–10; in Japan, 23, 39; job loss following, 80, 86–87; leakage from, 99; loss of identity following, 87–89; mammograms affected by, 37–38, 110–11; Mayo Clinic study of risk, 134–35, 140, 142–43; minimizing of symptoms associated with, 85–86, 115–44; misdiagnosis of symptoms associated with, 128–34; misinforming women of risks associated with, 91–114; the plastic surgeon's role in decision, 57–62; polyurethane-foam-covered, 29–32; psychiatric implications of, 25–27; reasons for choosing, 2–3, 9; as reconstructive surgery, 62–69, 100–105, 148–57; reformulation of, 32–37; relationships as influence on decision, 47–55, 172; removal of, 12, 161–63, 174–80; risk of infection, 37; risks associated with, 37–41, 71, 91–114; risks to children, 40–41, 79; rupture of, 4, 15–16, 33, 94, 111, 118–19, 121–22, 127; scientific evidence regarding risk, 37–41, 134–41, 142–44, 168; secrecy associated with, 75–76, 85–86, 163; self-esteem as issue in decision, 52–54, 55–57, 73–74; support groups for women with, 14–16, 84, 146–47, 167–68; surgical procedure, 20–21;

breast implants, silicone: (*continued*)
    symptoms associated with, 3–5, 12, 16,
    79–84, 115–17, 120, 121, 128–31, 139–
    40, 141–44, 148–49; uncertainties associ-
    ated with, 6–7, 19, 91, 187; women's re-
    sponses to, 73–78, 141–44, 145–68, 169–
    70; women's suspicions regarding, 164–66
breast injections, 21, 22, 23–24
breasts: importance of, to women, 5, 47–51,
    178–79
breast size: as medical issue, 6, 42–46
Bristol-Myers Squibb, 31, 108
Brown, Phil, 147–48
Brownmiller, Susan, 5, 50–51
Burton, Thomas, 140–41

capsular contracture, 37, 91, 119, 122
Chapkis, Wendy, 76
children: breast implants as risk to, 40–41,
    111–12
chronic fatigue, 4, 142
chronic fatigue syndrome, 12, 130
Clagette, D. T., 24
closed capsulotomy, 106, 118–19, 120
connective-tissue disease: associated with
    breast implants, 39, 136–37
Conway, Herbert, 24–25
Cook, Linda, 104–5
Cook, Robert, 12
cosmetic surgery: feminist debates on, 43–
    46. *See also* breast implants, silicone; plas-
    tic surgeons
Cronin, Thomas, 28–29, 33

Dalkon Shield, 132
Davis, Kathy, 43–45, 47, 71, 73, 76, 89, 90,
    169–70, 171
DES Action, 157
diethylstilbestrol (DES), 126, 132, 157–58
Doda, Carol, 23, 27
Dow Corning Corporation: blame directed
    at, 145; breast implant marketed by, 29;
    and reformulation of implants, 32; silicone
    developed by, 22, 28; lawsuits against, 2,
    32, 36–37, 140
Dull, Diana, 47, 56

Edgerton, M. T., 25
Ehrenreich, Barbara, 131
English, Deirdre, 131

Face to Face with Connie Chung: program on
    breast implants, 35–36, 115, 122
fatigue, 3
Fausto-Sterling, Anne, 125
femininity: cultural assumptions about, 5–6,
    44–46, 52, 89–90, 93, 96–100, 112–14,
    117–18, 172, 179; and removal of breast
    implants, 176–77
feminist perspectives: on cosmetic surgery,
    43–46
fibromyalgia, 12, 154
Food and Drug Administration (FDA): regu-
    lation of breast implants, 30, 97, 107–10;
    regulation of silicone use, 27–28; restric-
    tions on breast implants imposed by, 2, 6,
    14, 21, 31–32, 34–35, 140
Foucault, Michel, 45

Garfinkle, Harold, 135
gender. *See* femininity
Gerow, Frank, 28
Gordon, Deborah, 124–25
Goulian, Dicran, 24–25
Grindlay, J. H., 24

hair loss, 4, 91, 142
Hay, G. G., 26–27
health care system. *See* medical care system;
    plastic surgeons
Heyer-Schulte Corporation, 30–31
holistic health care, 155
Hopkins, Mariann, 2, 35
hot flashes, 16

implant mammaplasty. *See* breast implants
informed consent forms, 109–10
insurance: coverage for breast implants, 9–10
International Society of Plastic Surgeons,
    28–29
irritable bowel syndrome, 152
Ivalon, 24, 25

Jacobson, W. E., 27
joint pain, 4
Jones, Jenny, 36

Keller, Evelyn Fox, 136
Kessler, David, 35
Kumagai, Yauo, 39

La Leche League International, 40
Lappé, Marc, 138, 139
lawsuits: following breast implant surgery, 2, 32, 36–37, 140
Lloyd, Marilyn, 143
Lorde, Audre, 62, 64
lupus. *See* systemic lupus erythematosus

McClary, A. R., 25–26
mammograms: accuracy of affected by breast implants, 37–38, 110–11
Martin, Emily, 97, 125, 126
mastectomy: aftermath of, 148–57; reconstructive surgery following, 62–69, 100–105
Mayo Clinic: study on implant-related risk 134–35, 140, 142–43
medical care system: assumptions about, 92–93, 112–13, 185, 187; blamed for implant-related problems, 101–2, 146; fallibility of, 185–89; interaction with cultural assumptions about gender, 124–27; political-economic critiques of, 93–98
Medical Engineering Corporation, 108
medicalization, 42–43; damaging consequences of, 131–32
Menninger, Karl, 26
menopause, 126
menstruation, 126
methodology of study, 5–14, 17–18; demographics of respondents, 10–12
Meyer, E., 27
micromastia, 6, 25, 42
Mishler, Elliot, 147
Morgen, Sandra, 173

Oakley, Ann, 17–18

plastic surgeons: breast implant surgery as viewed by, 6, 8, 59–62, 98–100, 105–7, 178–79; risks minimized by, 93–96, 109
plastic surgery. *See* cosmetic surgery; breast implants, silicone
Pointer, Sam C., Jr., 36
polyurethane-foam-covered implants, 29–32
polyvinyl alcohol, 24
Prime Time Live: segment on breast implants, 4, 141
Public Citizen Research Group, 33, 137

reconstructive surgery: breast implants as, 62–69, 100–105, 148–57
relationships: impact of surgery on, 180–84; as influence on decision to have breast implants, 47–55, 172
rheumatic disorders, 115, 119, 170
rheumatoid arthritis, 4
Rothman, Barbara Katz, 112
Ruzek, Sheryl, 132

Sakurai, Dr., 23
Science on Trial: The Clash of Medical Evidence and the Law in the Breast Implant Case (Angell), 14, 139–40
scleroderma, 12, 87
Scottfoam Industrial Corporation, 31
self-esteem: as issue in decision to have breast implants, 52–54, 55–57, 73–74
sexuality: as affected by breast implant surgery, 16
silicone: injection of, into breasts, 22, 23–24; medical applications for, 22
Sjögren's syndrome, 12, 39, 87
sponges: Ivalon, 24–25; used as breast implants, 21
Stern, Maria, 32
support groups, 14–16, 84, 146–47, 167–68; on the Internet, 14
Surgitek, 31
systemic lupus erythematosus, 12, 39

Talcott, Tom, 33, 34
TDA (toluene diamine), 31
Todd, Alexandra Dundas, 92, 126
toluene diamine, 31

UpdeGraff, Howard, 26

Vasey, Frank, 137–38, 139

West, Candace, 47, 56
Wolfe, Sidney, 33, 137
World Wide Web: support groups available through, 14

Young, Iris, 5